# TRUTH, LIES,
—— AND ——
# PUBLIC HEALTH

# TRUTH, LIES, —— AND —— PUBLIC HEALTH

## How We Are Affected When Science and Politics Collide

Madelon Lubin Finkel

PRAEGER

Westport, Connecticut
London

**Library of Congress Cataloging-in-Publication Data**

Finkel, Madelon Lubin, 1949–
    Truth, lies, and public health : how we are affected when science and politics
collide / Madelon Lubin Finkel.
       p. ; cm.
    Includes bibliographical references and index.
    ISBN-13: 978-0-275-99128-9 (alk. paper)
    ISBN-10: 0-275-99128-8 (alk. paper)
    1. Medical policy—United States. I. Title.
    [DNLM: 1. Health Policy—United States. 2. Biomedical Research—legislation &
jurisprudence—United States. 3. Communicable Disease Control—legislation &
jurisprudence—United States. 4. Politics—United States. 5. Public Health—legislation &
jurisprudence—United States. WA 540 AA1 F499t 2007]
    RA395.A3F537   2007
    362.10973—dc22        2007016345

British Library Cataloguing in Publication Data is available.

Library of Congress Catalog Card Number: 2007016345
ISBN-13: 978-0-275-99128-9
ISBN-10: 0-275-99128-8

First published in 2007

Praeger Publishers, 88 Post Road West, Westport, CT 06881
An imprint of Greenwood Publishing Group, Inc.
www.praeger.com

Printed in the United States of America

The paper used in this book complies with the
Permanent Paper Standard issued by the National
Information Standards Organization (Z39.48–1984).

10  9  8  7  6  5  4  3  2  1

For Arnold
thank you for your support, advice, and love

# Contents

# Preface

People in general have no notion of the sort and the amount of evidence often needed to prove the simplest matter of fact.

Peter Mere Latham, MD (1789–1875)

As an epidemiologist who also has a keen interest in health care policy, I have often been struck firstly by how hard it is to conduct a bias-free study, and secondly how easy it is to take the findings of a study and interpret the findings to suit one's purposes. Obtaining valid and reliable findings is so dependent on the study population, the study design, and the study methodology. That being said, what a scientist hopes to accomplish by his or her research is to provide a greater sense of clarity of the issue based on the data. What a scientist wants to avoid is the distortion of the findings to suit a particular political position. The data should speak for themselves and should be based on an objective (that is, apolitical) premise. Of course, there are legitimate differences of opinion about many issues, regardless of study findings. In particular, those studies that focus on social and ethical issues, in which one could expect to see legitimate differences of opinion, often generate the most intense debate.

All too often, we have heard of examples of research studies being used to provide evidence for one point of view or other. And, as history has shown, there are many instances in which research findings are so clear and so compelling yet policy decision making was based on a majority party's political position regardless of the evidence. The politicalization of science has a long history and is not unique to one particular political party. At times, however, these political decisions can be harmful to society. More often than not had policy been based on the evidence, diseases that could have been kept in check or even have been eliminated ended up infecting large numbers of people.

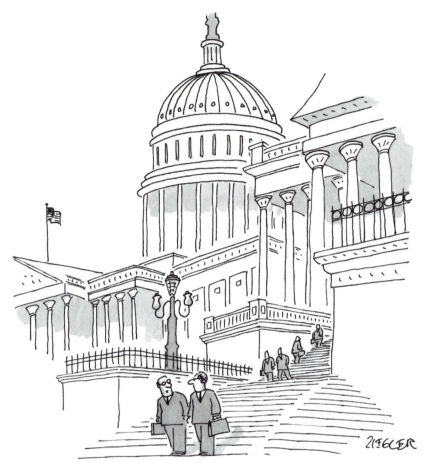

*"Of course it would be a different story entirely if we could extract crude oil from stem cells."*

The essays in this book have been written to make a point: the politicalization of science is a slippery slope and can end up doing more harm than good. Each of the topics was carefully selected primarily because there are research findings available that should have been used to guide policy making. In an ideal world, regardless of one's personal perspective of the issue, the body of evidence available should have trumped any political distortion of the facts. In reality, however, ideological politics often trumped the science. Each essay includes a brief history of the issues as background to the current political situation. Each focuses on the social, economic, ethical, and political components of the issue (when applicable). Different sides of the issue are presented, although in some cases the writer's bias may be evident. It also must be said that many of the issues discussed in the book are currently being debated. As such, new information is constantly being published; new laws are being enacted; in short, policy is evolving. The material in each chapter, however, is the most current as of early 2007.

## POLITICS AND SCIENCE

Pretending that politics and science do not coexist is foolish, and cleanly separating science from politics is probably neither feasible nor recommended. Indeed, most scientists and politicians would advocate that science should be relevant to policy. What one needs to guard against, however, is science and public health policy being dictated by ideology. Policy makers should strive for an honest interpretation of scientific findings, which then would drive the formulation of policy making. Independent and critical thinking contributes to the dynamic dialogue; muzzling those whose views are at odds with the majority party or distorting evidence to fit one's point of view is not only bad science, but also bad politics. Policy, it should be said, is also compromised when it is solely determined by science at the exclusion of social, cultural, and ethical considerations.

For better or worse, politics is an important and influential forum in which policy is shaped. Most of the significant advances in public health policy, for example, can be made only in the context of a political debate. Each of the essays relate to a politically supercharged topic. Not surprisingly, then, policy debates often have been motivated by narrow political agendas that may or may not have been based on the available scientific evidence. Discussion about how best to protect the public is often an afterthought, and using the available data honestly and objectively to support one's position also is often an afterthought. What we have seen time and time again, alas, is the lack of restraint of political considerations in light of clear and convincing scientific evidence. The issue is not to insulate public health research from politics, rather how to use research and the scientific process more effectively to educate and guide the politics of public health.

The topics included in this book reflect the delicate trade-offs between private rights and public goods. In many instances, personal values may clash with scientific findings. To what extent, then, should public policy be reflective of personal values? The difficulty, indeed the danger, lies in shaping public policy in absence or disregard of objective, quality research. Chapter 1 focuses on the uneasy partnership of politics and science and argues that political ideology must take a backseat to empirical evidence in formulating science/public health policy. A brief history of science-based policy in the United States is presented, including the role of the scientific advisory committee system. Examples of science policy making under recent Presidents illustrate that both the Democratic and the Republican parties have used politics to shape science policy, but that President George W. Bush, in particular, has taken what one could argue is a politically extreme partisan political position in setting public health and science policy. Using ideology or political considerations to set policy, and then seeking scientific justification for it, diminishes and discredits the scientific political process. The chapter concludes with a plea for protecting the independent integrity of the scientific process and for guarding against the politicalization of setting science policy. Rather than pretending that politics and science do not coexist, a better course of action is to try to develop a transparent and accountable system to neutralize the danger of politics trampling the scientific process.

## THE POLITICS OF CONTRACEPTION

The intermingling of politics with the most private and personal act of contraception has had a long and troubled history in the United States. Women's reproductive health has been a lightening rod for politicians of every stripe to take a stand, in some cases irrespective of the potential danger to the woman's health. Social conservatives, in particular, have long opposed government efforts to support birth control both for adults and especially for adolescents. Throughout the long history of finding ways to control fertility, strong moral sentiments, religious beliefs, legal constraints, and gender relations often limited the provision of advice and methods of birth control. Victorian values, sexual prudishness, moral objections to birth control, and political gamesmanship often made it difficult or impossible to obtain and use safe and effective contraception. In addition to the religious and moral beliefs limiting the availability of contraception, economic barriers also prevented (and to a certain extent still prevent) many women from obtaining safe and effective methods of birth control.

Chapter 2 focuses on this highly contentious issue by providing a historical overview showing how safe contraception has contributed to one of the twentieth century's most dramatic social revolutions: the redefinition of roles and opportunities for women. The essay discusses the ideological views on contraceptive practices in light of scientific findings. The clash between science, religion, and politics is a constant theme in the provision of safe, legal, and effective contraception in the United States. Yet, perhaps the most egregious example of the disregard of the scientific evidence to achieve a political aim surrounds the debate over the legal availability of Plan B, the morning after pill. The controversy over Plan B highlights how issues can get highjacked by the political process and undermine decades of judicial rulings and legislative acts. Despite the significant body of research showing the safety, efficacy, and cost-effectiveness of contraception in general and Plan B in particular; despite the empirical evidence showing that over the counter access to emergency contraception improves women's lives and health by preventing unintended, or unwanted pregnancies; and despite the fact that it is safer to take Plan B, for example, than to have an abortion or to carry the pregnancy to term, the access to and availability of emergency contraception was being severely limited by those whose personal beliefs were contrary to the dissemination of this particular drug. The FDA's shameful stalling and its disregard for the law and its own principles only serves to illustrate what can occur when science is trampled by politics. The conclusion drawn by the author is that by caving in to ideology rather than evidence, the FDA's handling of Plan B has tarnished its image and compromised its reputation as an objective scientific agency.

## THE POLITICS OF HIV/AIDS

Early in the HIV/AIDS epidemic, the lack of knowledge about this new and deadly infection hampered the ability to design policy. Confounding the issue was *who* (which population groups) was getting sick. HIV/AIDS was a terrifying disease that was made more complicated by the political handling of it. Perhaps millions of lives could have been saved had political action been taken in a more timely manner. It took years for the government to appreciate the seriousness of the growing crisis both in the United States and abroad. Indeed, it was the private sector that led the charge on dealing with the epidemic. Chapter 3 focuses on the pandemic AIDS epidemic and the interplay between science, politics, and economics. A comprehensive historical review helps define the issues and explains how the world got itself in the present state. The point that hopefully is made in this essay is that from the beginning of the epidemic, AIDS was a controversial, politically charged issue that made class, race, gender, socioeconomic, and geographic inequities painfully obvious. Fear, stigma, ignorance, and apathy about AIDS increased human rights violations against people living with HIV/AIDS, and human rights violations facilitated the spread of AIDS.

Today, there fortunately has been progress made in terms of treating those who are HIV positive and those who have full-blown AIDS. But, there still remains so much to do in terms of treatment, prevention, and education. Less than ten years after the development of the "cocktail" of drugs now widely used to treat AIDS in many developed nations, only a small percentage of those in Africa and Asia who need the drugs have access to them. The single most important impediment is the exorbitantly high cost of the medications. What happens in the future depends very much on what the international community does now. It will be increasingly harder to sustain treatment programs unless we can dramatically reduce the number of new HIV infections. Much more needs to be done in the area of prevention.

## THE POLITICS OF STEM CELL RESEARCH

Few areas of biomedical science have aroused as much controversy as embryonic stem cell research. Since the derivation of the first human embryonic stem cells in 1998, the issue has been at the forefront of scientific, ethical, and political debates. Proponents of stem cell research emphasize the considerable therapeutic potential, including the possibility of curing a wide range of diseases. Stem cells appear to offer unprecedented opportunities for developing new medical therapies for many debilitating diseases and a new way to explore fundamental questions of biology. Physicians, scientists, and those in business envision tremendous economic benefits of a burgeoning stem cell industry, just as individuals with incurable diseases envision the medical miracles that could possibly help them. On the other hand, opponents of stem cell research speak of the immorality of utilizing human cells. At the crux of this debate is the issue of an embryo's "personhood." With so many important and controversial sides to this debate, it would be ideal to have a rational and coherent national dialogue; however, in reality, the ethical and religious aspect of the issue is making it difficult to reach an agreement or compromise regarding stem cell research.

Chapter 4 focuses on the ethical, political, and scientific issues surrounding the stem cell controversy. Because embryonic stem cells have the potential to grow into any tissue or organ in the body, scientists believe that they hold great promise for treatment and cures. But, because human embryos are destroyed in extracting the stem cells, there are intense objections from abortion opponents. The bitter debate surrounding embryonic stem cell research took an interesting turn after the November 2006 election. The Democrats gained control of Congress and drafted legislation to loosen President George W. Bush's restrictions on federal support of embryonic stem cell research. The Democrats' bill would expand the number of embryonic cell lines by including human embryonic stem cells regardless of when they were derived (i.e., from surplus embryos that were originally created for fertility treatments and would otherwise be discarded). The Bush administration is opposed to this bill. Time will tell in which direction the United States will go regarding embryonic stem cell research.

## SCIENCE, POLITICS, AND MEDICAL MARIJUANA

The history of the legitimate and legal medical uses of marijuana clearly shows how political ideology, rhetoric, and action impeded, in fact made almost impossible, scientific quantification of the risks and benefits of marijuana (Cannabis). Cannabis has been used for medicinal purposes for thousands of years. Chapter 5 provides a colorful history of the medical use of marijuana. Over the past decades, legal and legislative actions highlight the twisted path of the legal use of marijuana for medical purposes. Legislation made very little distinction between narcotics, cocaine, and marijuana; federal law did not recognize any distinction between marijuana and other illicit substances. In fact, the U.S. federal government does not, and never has, recognized legitimate medical uses of marijuana.

While the 1937 Marijuana Tax Act effectively stopped physicians from using marijuana as medicine, the 1970 Controlled Substances Act placed marijuana as a Schedule I drug and subsequent efforts to move marijuana from Schedule I to another schedule repeatedly failed. Whereas the option of pre-scribing and using marijuana for medical purposes was blocked by court decree, physicians can prescribe morphine and other narcotics. Unlike many other psychoactive drugs, marijuana now cannot be prescribed to patients even in cases where physicians believe that it would be beneficial. The reasons for this prohibition are clearly politically ideological, but what was the basis for this ideology?

While the federal policy toward marijuana clearly made little distinction between narcotics, cocaine, and marijuana, individual states took, and continue to take, a more liberal view of marijuana. For example, numerous states allow for the medical use of marijuana. This essay examines the scientific evidence for and against the use of marijuana for medical purposes and discusses the 2005 Supreme Court ruling on the legalization of medical marijuana. A ruling against the federal government would have had far-reaching legal implications but also would have been a major blow to the aggressive George W. Bush White House antimarijuana policies. In a stinging 6–3 defeat against the proponents of medical marijuana, the court ruling continued to put the federal government at odds with many in the scientific community and with public opinion. What the case didn't do is settle the question of whether marijuana is an effective medi-cine. The scientific evidence is presented for the reader to come to his or her own conclusion.

## THE POLITICS OF NEEDLE EXCHANGE PROGRAMS

The history of needle exchange programs (NEPs), particularly in the United States, is a clear example of how politics can run roughshod over science. Even though the scientific research uniformly showed that providing clean nee-dles to injection drug users is an effective means of reducing the spread of HIV and hepatitis C virus, barriers to developing such exchange programs effectively prevented this public health measure from being implemented on a wide scale. In Chapter 6, we discuss the story behind the federal ban for fund-ing NEPs and the implications of this policy.

Today, four presidential administrations and five surgeon generals later, the 12-year-old federal funding ban of NEPs continues to be in effect. The United States remains the only country in the world to directly oppose the scienti-fically proven cost-effective intervention in preventing HIV and AIDS. The federal ban in funding NEPs, coupled with reluctance of most politicians in Washington, DC, to take a controversial stance, has left NEPs across the nation struggling. The polarized debate of the pros and cons of NEPs continues to stymie U.S. federal policy. Individual states have taken action, but there is lit-tle uniformity in law among them. Some would argue that the time is long overdue to separate the War on Drugs from the War on AIDS. To do anything otherwise would be unethical, discriminatory, and irresponsible.

## THE POLITICS OF TB CONTROL

TB continues to pose a huge threat to global health and is today still one of the world's most serious infectious diseases. The history of the rise and fall, and again rise, in TB is a sad, yet instructive one. TB is preventable and treatable, and there is a cost-effective cure for this disease, which is not the case for many other infectious diseases. TB it is a political as much as a medical problem—and so are the solutions. It just depends on how much governments are prepared to spend. Apathy, complacency, funding cuts, and lack of access to treatment, individually and collectively, helped create the situation we face today. Ironically, unlike other deadly infectious diseases, TB more often than not responds quickly and effectively to treatment. Chapter 7 provides a historical overview to TB control measures and discusses how political apathy led to not only a resurgence in this once dreaded disease but also to the situation we now face: multidrug resistant strains of TB.

The history of TB control provides a cautionary tale to those entrusted to safeguard the health of the public. As history has shown, ignoring the reality that TB is a major infectious disease worldwide is dangerous; an untreated person with active TB can infect others quite easily. Point in fact, inadequate TB control now appears to be a major cause of multidrug-resistant TB (MDR-TB). MDR-TB is a form of TB that is resistant to two or more of the primary drugs used for the treatment of TB. Clearly, the success of treatment depends upon how quickly a case of TB is identified as drug resistant and whether an effective drug therapy is available. It is well known that multidrug-resistant strains of TB are not only more difficult to treat, but they are also more costly and deadly; the case fatality is extremely high as the overwhelming majority of those with MDR-TB die relatively quickly.

While MDR-TB is certainly alarming, very recently a new and extremely dangerous form of TB has been identified: a "virtually untreatable" form of TB has now emerged. Extreme drug resistant TB (XDR-TB) has been seen worldwide, including the United States, Eastern Europe, and Africa. XDR-TB, in addition to the two first-line drugs used to treat TB, is also resistant to three or more of the six classes of second-line drugs. What makes this strain of TB so lethal is that XDR-TB can infect even the healthiest of people. While the chance of survival is greater among healthy people because these individuals are more likely to be able to fight off the disease, those who have compromised immune systems due to HIV and AIDS who develop XDR-TB usually will die within a month. The outlook is not very pretty at all.

## SCIENCE, POLITICS, AND THE REGULATION OF DIETARY SUPPLEMENTS

The dietary supplement industry would have the public believe that supplements can help stave off disease, improve one's energy level, and that they are safe. In some cases, their claims are correct. In other cases, the epidemiological evidence is not as clearcut or as positive. Given that so many people consume one or more dietary supplements on a regular basis, there is growing concern about the efficacy and safety of these products, which are readily and easily available for purchase over-the-counter in supermarkets, drug stores, health food stores, and on the Internet.

Chapter 8 focuses on the dietary supplement industry. For years, millions of Americans have spent billions of dollars on alternative remedies whose benefits and risks have not been rigorously studied. Supplements are often perceived as safe because they are "natural"; but what the public needs to understand is that many dietary supplements can and do have a powerful effect on the body. This chapter reviews the epidemiological evidence for many of the popular dietary supplements (vitamins and herbals, in particular) and discusses federal policy regarding the regulation of these products. It will be shown how the dietary supplement industry has consistently and strongly resisted effective federal regulation and has used its considerable political and economic clout to make sure its wishes were respected. Legislation passed in the twentieth century largely ignored or exempted dietary supplements from effective oversight and regulation. The most striking example of the laissez-faire attitude towards the dietary supplement industry is best illustrated by the passage of the Dietary Supplement Health and Education Act of 1994 (DSHEA), which is now the primary framework for the regulation of dietary supplements.

## SILICONE BREAST IMPLANTS: MISCONCEPTIONS, MISINTERPRETATIONS, AND MISTAKES

Essentially, the silicone breast implant saga illustrates how the American legal system failed to meet the challenge of separating scientific facts from anecdotal testimony, and how difficult it was for juries to differentiate scientifically valid evidence from "junk" science and emotionally laden personal stories. The lessons to be learned from this emotionally charged issue are many, but the one that supersedes the others is that the scientific approach to assessing risk and causality must take precedent in the courtroom.

Chapter 9 focuses on the silicone gel breast implant controversy and pieces together the complex scientific and legal issues that are so central to the case. An in-depth review of the epidemiological evidence is presented along with the legal court rulings. The silicone gel breast implant story highlights the dangers of permitting unscientific studies to be introduced into the courts. Without proper scientific evidence, finding a party guilty or liable violates the spirit of the law and undermines the purpose of the legal system. However, as was evident in the early court cases, judges and juries often did not know what was considered valid testimony or valid scientific evidence. To ensure that the scientific evidence proffered was not based on personal opinions, the courts, over the years, have tried to set standards upon which expert testimony must be assessed.

## THE POLITICS OF OBESITY

Americans are the fattest people on earth. How Americans achieved this dubious distinction can partially be understood by examining the economics and politics of the food industry. Chapter 10 focuses on the causes and consequences of obesity, as well as the economics and politics associated with it. The main debate between "personal responsibility" and "public interest" is complex and contentious. Compounding the issue is that most people do not consider being fat a disease. They see overweight and obesity as a lifestyle problem. Many are confused by the changing food pyramid guidelines, the ever-changing list of foods to eat and not to eat, and celebrity diet crazes. Added to all this is the daily bombardment of advertisements for inexpensive and plentiful fast food options. The obesity epidemic has reached the point where even McDonald's, the purveyor of Big Macs and super-sized portions of French fries, is throwing its weight behind obesity research, as well as the promotion of what it calls balanced, active lifestyles.

Given that the science is clear about the causes and correlates of overweight and obesity, what is the government's policy to help stem this epidemic? What are the economics and politics of obesity? What has been the food industry's response to the situation? There is no equivalent to "Don't Smoke" or "Just Say No to Drugs." U.S. food policy is reviewed and programs designed to promote healthier eating are presented. The issue is not how social and environmental change can occur in the current political climate, but how politics in the future (public policy) can contribute to social and environmental change.

## DISEASE PREVENTION THROUGH VACCINATION: THE SCIENCE AND THE CONTROVERSY

Vaccinations have largely eliminated once-common, terrible diseases such as polio, measles, smallpox, and diphtheria. In the United States, politics has contributed to successful public health policies by requiring vaccination at school entry, which has been vital in achieving high vaccine coverage in children. But, the path to disease eradication has not always been smooth. In addition to the scientific challenges to vaccine development, social, ethical, economic, legal, and political issues individually and collectively have served to curtail and in some cases to derail efforts to immunize populations. Vociferous antivaccination movements frequently clashed with the government's authority to immunize for the "common good." Historically, antivaccinationists have protested against what they consider the intrusion of their privacy and bodily integrity.

Chapter 11 focuses on vaccine policies, vaccine controversies, and the very current debate over the human papilloma virus (HPV) vaccine. At issue is Gardasil, a three-dose vaccine developed by Merck and Co. and approved by the FDA in 2006. The vaccine protects against strains of the human papilloma virus that account for an estimated 70% of the cases of cervical cancer and genital warts. Perhaps the most contentious issue of HPV vaccination is the recommendation to vaccinate young girls and women between the ages of eleven and twenty-six. Social conservative religious groups have publicly opposed the concept of making HPV vaccination mandatory for preadolescent girls because they fear that this might send a subtle message that sexual intercourse is okay, thus detracting from their abstinence-based position. Other critics question *mandating* the vaccine for young girls. Many parents are extremely uncomfortable at the notion of vaccinating their young daughters against a sexually transmitted disease. But the reality is that the vaccine will not work after a woman has been infected, so the thinking is that it is preferable to have the young girl vaccinated before she becomes sexually active. Not surprisingly, there is heated debate as to whether the vaccinations should be required or recommended. Proponents argue that the objections are not strong enough to forgo the protection against a potentially dangerous disease. Although Texas is the only state so far to mandate the vaccine, other states are considering doing so. However, these states will have to make their decision without the heavy lobbying from Merck. Merck agreed to stop lobbying state legislatures to require the use of its new vaccine.

The success of immunization policies depends on, and is linked with, interrelated factors including vaccine safety (quality control and monitoring); adequate vaccine supply (to avoid vaccine shortages); effective delivery systems to insure that the vaccines get to those in need (more of an issue in the developing world); financial incentives and legal protection for the vaccine manufacturers; and educational efforts to inform the public about the benefits and risks of vaccinations. Indeed, perhaps most of all, there is a need to focus on the public's fears about the safety of vaccination and their willingness to be immunized.

## CONCLUSION

For many things in life, most of us do not know much about what is risky and what isn't. Much of what we think we understand comes from the media, who may or may not be interpreting the findings of scientific studies correctly. Indeed, journalists, and even the researchers themselves, are partly responsible for the way health risks are inflated or distorted in the media. Complicating this issue is the fact that findings from epidemiological studies can differ depending on who is included in the study, how the study was designed, how long the study was conducted, and so forth. There are legitimate reasons for inconsistent or even contrary findings. Add to this mix the politics of an issue and we have a very meaty stew. What is important is to guard against the introduction of politics to achieve a partisan aim. Manipulating research findings to support one's position is a dishonest way to formulate policy. Ignoring conclusive evidence because it does not support one's position is also a counterproductive way to formulate policy. Debate is important, but it should be based on the facts, the evidence, not on opinions or hearsay.

The essays in this book tried to illustrate the potential danger in the use, misuse, and misinterpretation of science in the formulation of public policy. By taking a historical perspective to better understand the issues, one can appreciate and maybe even understand how public policy was made.

# Acknowledgments

I consider myself to be the luckiest of individuals because I have the support and encouragement of so many people. As a medical school professor at one of the top medical schools in the country, I have access to so many bright and accomplished students. Their interest in the book and their willingness to help research the topics made the writing of the chapters so much more fun and interesting for me. In many respects, this book is a product of collaborative efforts and discussion. As a way of thanking my students for taking the time out of their busy medical school schedule to research a topic that they found interesting, I am pleased to include their names as contributor to the specific chapter. Thank you Ryan Cauley, Sandra Demars, Ivan Ip, MPH, Joanna Paladino, and Tony Rosen, MPH. Thanks also to Jennifer Swails who conducted the initial research on dietary supplements.

Thank you to my editor, Debbie Carvalko, who provided the encouragement for the writing of this book and who never lost faith that the manuscript would be delivered to her.

Thanks also to the politicians who more often than not took the information and molded it to reflect what they wanted to believe. Without them, this book would be unnecessary.

Most of all, I give thanks to the scientists who spend their years conducting research in an effort to provide us with facts and truths. Without them, our ability to implement public health policy would be seriously limited.

# —— 1 ——

# About Politics and Science

Science advising in government is unavoidably political, but we must make a concerted effort to ensure that it is democratic.[1]

Perhaps it is naïve to assume that politics and science are separate and distinct fields of interest never to intrude on or interfere with the other. Perhaps it is naïve to assume that policy makers would want to base their decisions on the best possible evidence, regardless of their political leanings. In a perfect world, I suppose all policy decisions would be made based on research and hypothesis testing, but we in the United States are not living in a utopian, apolitical society and in many matters, particularly the thorny social/ethical issues of the time, politics and science are intertwined. Pretending that politics and science do not coexist is foolish, and cleanly separating science from politics is probably neither feasible nor recommended. Indeed, most scientists and politicians would advocate that science should be relevant to policy. What one needs to guard against, however, is permitting a political agenda to dictate the scientific process. Policy makers should strive for an honest interpretation of scientific findings, which then would drive the formulation of policy making. What we have seen time and time again, alas, is the lack of restraint of political considerations in light of clear and convincing scientific evidence.

Science policy and public policy are necessarily interconnected, but inherent in this symbiotic relationship lies distinct differences in approach. In science, facts are a reality. In politics, perceptions and interpretations of facts are a reality. Facts are negotiable and policy making is based on competing interests, conflicting objectives, and trade-offs, which often can lead to a conscious or unconscious selectivity in interpreting facts to shape policy. Often, those engaged in political issues try to gain an advantage over their opponents by influencing the availability and perception of information to increase the odds of a favorable outcome. Science policy decision making as well as federal funding for scientific research, which is in the billions of dollars, is often at the mercy of politics.

It is important to draw a distinction between science *politics* and science *policy*. From a *political perspective*, science has often been used to reduce choice among decision makers to a preferred outcome that reflects political positions on specific issues. In contrast, a *science policy perspective* should focus on using scientific findings to *guide* decision makers in policy planning.[2] While politicians rely on scientific evidence to make their case for or against an issue, scientists and researchers, who are supposed to be above the political fray, should be the protectors of scientific findings and should guard against nonscientists distorting their findings in an effort to seek desired political outcomes. Often, both sides are relying on the same information and seeking to "spin" the latest scientific findings to favor their position. While the data are usually the same, it is the interpretation of the data that can get lost in the political battle.

David H. Guston, in his book *Between Politics and Science*, examines the complex relationship between science and politics in an intelligent and interesting manner.[3] His historical perspective illustrates how inexorably entwined the two have become. He writes, "Policy in science involves the direction of funds; science in policy involves the provision of expertise from science to politics."[4]

Science policy making involves the allocation of funds to "worthy" projects, but the interpretation of "worthy" often is made within a political context that at times belies scientific merit. The uneasy relationship between politics and science also has been examined by Howard J. Silver, who takes a prospective view on the issue, explaining that as scientific discoveries and advances create ethical dilemmas (stem cell research, cloning, nanotechnology, and the like), the political intrusion will certainly grow.[5] In *Politicizing Science: The Alchemy of Policymaking*, a collection of essays written by eleven leading scientists and edited by biologist Michael Gough, the authors describe how the consequences of politicalization are inflicted on the public, including the diversion of money and research efforts, the costs of unnecessary regulations, and the manipulation of scientific funding to advance a policy agenda.[6] The authors imply that money goes a long way toward explaining complaints over the politicization of science. That is, once government funds science, and since World War II it has funded approximately 50% of all science research, the funding decisions can become political, to say the least. These authors sound the alarm that science is losing its independent, apolitical position in society.

## GETTING PERSONAL: THE POLITICALIZATION OF THE SCIENCE ADVISOR

For hundreds of years, scientific advances in all fields of study have shaped, defined, and transformed society. During the twentieth century, where billions of federal dollars were spent on research in virtually every field of scientific endeavor, discoveries in the realm of space exploration, the physical sciences, and the biological/medical sciences transcended political dictates for the most part. Today, new frontiers in genome and nanotechnology, stem cell research, and molecular biology, for example, hold great promise for further discoveries and advances. But these new areas of research, made possible by the scientific advances of the past, often embody thorny social and ethical issues that, at times, have sparked vociferous and contentious debate. Sorting out competing scientific claims, ethical dilemmas, and political needs makes the policy-makers' task of implementing public policy that much harder. Charges of a politicization of science, even a disregard for scientific evidence, have heightened the tensions between the scientific and political communities. In the past, for example, a scientist's personal political beliefs were not used as a litmus test to receive federal funding; however, today, political ideology seems to have become an important consideration. The erosion of scientific integrity has been accelerated under the Bush II administration, but certainly existed to some degree in some form under other presidents.

Scientists since Benjamin Franklin have been acting as advisors to the government, and as such, played active roles in policy making. History shows that presidents have sought the advice of scientists regardless of the individual's party affiliation. The objective was to get the best minds together during the policy-making process. It was President Eisenhower who first officially created the position of science advisor, perhaps propelled to do so by the Russian's success with Sputnik. He appointed the best minds to serve on the Science Advisory Committee. President Kennedy, too, sought out scientists into the highest councils of government, and one's party affiliation was not a consideration. The belief was that science and scientists were above politics. As Daniel Greenberg wrote in his book, *Science, Money, Politics*, scientists might have considered themselves Republicans or Democrats, but as politicians saw it, science was their true party affiliation, and scientists saw it that way, too.[7]

During the 1950s, the Cold War years, the focus was on "winning" the space race against the Russians and eliminating infectious diseases (polio is a prime example). The goals were so clear that there was no clash between science and politics. Things began to get more complicated in the 1960s. The nation as a whole became more political (the Vietnam War was certainly a divisive force) and scientists, too, entered the political fray. During the presidential campaign of the mid-1960s, Barry Goldwater declared his willingness to deploy nuclear weapons on the battlefield. Scientists were vociferously against this position and formed a group called Scientists and Engineers for Johnson. This was probably the first time in history that a significant number of scientists, galvanized by politics, took a public stance in such a large way.

President Nixon clashed with scientists over the latter's opposition to the antiballistic missile system and other administration science programs. He actually tried to squelch research funding at the Massachusetts Institute of

Technology in retaliation against its president, who opposed missile defense. Nixon also reacted by abolishing the position of science advisor, as well as the Office of Science and Technology after the advisor failed to support Nixon's quest for a supersonic airplane. President Gerald Ford, upon assuming the presidency, reinstated this position, viewing it as an important advisory entity on science and technology matters.

Congress, of course, was actively involved in formulating science policy. In the mid-1970s, Congress passed the National Science and Technology Policy, Organization, and Priorities Act of 1976, which established a federal administrative organization for science policy and articulated a science policy for the nation. This act established the Office of Science and Technology Policy (OSTP), whose mission is to serve as a source of scientific and technological analysis and judgment for the President with respect to major policies, plans, and programs of the federal government. The OSTP is authorized to advise the president and others within the Executive Office of the President on the impacts of science and technology on domestic and international affairs. It also is to help develop and implement sound science and technology policies and budget, among other things.

The intermingling of science and politics intensified during the Reagan presidency. To a certain extent, partisan science disagreements began in the late 1980s when science and technology became politicized in Congress as part of a broader political strategy. Former House Speaker Newt Gingrich led the charge to fight Democrats on just about everything, including science policy. But, one of the most egregious acts of partisan science politics during this time actually backfired. When President Reagan nominated Dr. C. Everett Koop to the position of Surgeon General, it was well known that Dr. Koop was a staunch conservative. He also had no public health experience (he was a noted pediatric surgeon), but Reagan selected him in a blatant attempt to place ideology and ideological fealty over the needs and demands of the public. The battle over Koop's nomination dragged on for almost a year before he was finally approved. The religious and political right assumed that they had an ally as head of the Public Health Service, but Dr. Koop's scientific integrity trumped ideology, much to the chagrin of his supporters.

To fight the growing epidemic of acquired immunodeficiency syndrome (AIDS), Dr. Koop recommended a program of compulsory sex education in the schools, and he also argued that children should be taught how to use condoms. He was an ardent antismoking crusader, which angered the tobacco industry. When President Reagan asked him to prepare a report on the psychological effects of abortion, he did so in a scientific way meeting with individuals on both sides of the issue and reviewing hundreds of scientific publications. While the conservatives felt certain that Dr. Koop would see things their way, the evidence did not support that position and Dr. Koop declined to say that abortion was always more damaging than the alternative. He further declined to say that there wasn't enough data to support either side's position. The administration was shocked (and probably annoyed) at Dr. Koop's refusal to change his stance. Dr. Koop summed up the issue best when he said, "You know, I never changed my stripes during all that time, and I still haven't. What I did in that job was what any well-trained doctor or scientists would do: I looked at the data and then presented the facts to the American people. In science, you can't hide from the data."[8]

The challenge of assuring the integrity of science was forced into the limelight in the 1980s after allegations were made public about misconduct with respect to research supported by the National Cancer Institute. Then-Representative Al Gore and Senator Orin Hatch led a congressional investigation of scientific misconduct, and the upshot of these hearings was that research integrity could no longer be informally managed within the scientific community. Congress created the Office of Research Integrity (ORI) within the National Institutes of Health (NIH) and the Offices of the Inspector General within the National Science Foundation (NSF) to assist in assuring research integrity. ORI's focus on scientific misconduct was to ensure that research programs function within appropriate parameters to maintain federal funding. Congress also passed legislation to create the Office of Technology Transfer to facilitate the transfer of and remuneration for scientific discoveries among the public and private sectors, while also encouraging both the integrity and productivity of science.

The National Science and Technology Council (NSTC), established by an executive order on November 23, 1993, is a Cabinet-level council chaired by the President, whose principal mission is to coordinate science and technology policy across the diverse entities that make up the federal research and development enterprise. One of the primary objectives of the NSTC is the establishment of clear national goals for federal science and technology investments in a broad array of areas spanning virtually all the mission areas of the executive branch. The NSTC prepares research and development strategies that are coordinated across federal agencies to form investment packages aimed at accomplishing multiple national goals. The work of the NSTC is organized under four primary committees: Science, Technology, Environment and Natural Resources, and Homeland and National Security. Each of these committees oversees subcommittees and working groups focused on different aspects of science and technology and working to coordinate across the federal government. These federal entities serve to integrate science and public policy at the highest level of government.

## SCIENTIFIC ADVISORY COMMITTEES AND POLICY FORMULATION

In addition to the numerous federal agencies created to promote scientific research and to develop science-based policies (the NIH, Food and Drug Administration, Centers for Disease Control and Prevention [CDC], for example), there are hundreds of federal scientific advisory committees whose role is to advise the legislative and executive branches of the government on science matters. The Federal Advisory Committee Act of 1972 established uniform procedures for committees, which had to be specifically authorized by Congress, by the president, or by an agency head. All advisory committees must have written charters. The act also required committee membership to be fairly balanced in terms of points of view represented. These advisory committees play an important role in developing and guiding the federal government's science policy and are created to address scientific, technical, and medical issues. For many federal agencies, particularly those focusing on medicine and health, advisory committees are chartered to address the most challenging and contentious scientific issues. The committees are meant to provide independent, expert, and objective advice on policy and the funding of research. At times, advisory committees have not always reached consensus, but the differences debated contribute to the dialogue. The committees' recommendations are to be based on independent judgment and should not be inappropriately influenced by any special interest group or the appointing authority.

Advisory committees do not make decisions per se; their purpose is to advise. Nor were they created to tell the executive or legislative branch what they want to hear. Although Congress and the executive branch may ignore the advice given, such action should be based on the facts, not on politics. Consistent with federal law, the president and heads of departments and agencies have the right to choose the advisors they want. Politics surely plays a role in the selection of members of the committees, but it is quite inappropriate to staff an advisory board with people who hold the same (political) views about the issue. Stacking the boards to eliminate dissent goes against Congress' intent to ensure ideological diversity. An advisory board's recommendations should be based on independent judgment and should not be inappropriately influenced by special interest groups and the like. Of course, in the real world, this is not always the case.

What happens when the advisory committee system is manipulated for political and ideological purposes? When the political process uses science and scientists to further the party's political objectives, the presumed neutrality of science is jeopardized. Yet, as history has shown, both Republican and Democratic administrations have employed such tactics, some more egregiously than other, however. The Nixon administration, for example, was accused of politicalizing the advisory committee appointment process in its attempt to gain control over the NIH budget. During the Reagan administration, there was a controversy about a "hit list" of scientific advisors to the Environmental Protection Agency who were targeted for exclusion because of their liberal or pro-environment viewpoint.[9] President George Bush's administration (Bush I) was accused of questioning candidates for leading positions about their views on abortion. Dr. Louis Sullivan, the then Secretary of the Department of Health and Human Services, drew a line at the level of assistant secretary for health saying below that level there would be no ideological litmus test.[10]

As the pressing public health issues became more socially and ethically oriented, the politicalization of science intensified. President Clinton refused to lift the ban on needle exchange programs despite evidence that clean needles would do much to stop the spread of human immunodeficiency virus (HIV), AIDS, and other diseases and despite the urging by scientific advisors to do so. The head of the NIH, his own Secretary of Health and Human Services, and his Drug Czar also advocated in support of needle exchange programs to stem the spread of disease. Clinton later acknowledged that his decision was counter that of his scientific advisors and that his decision was politically driven.

Toward the end of the twentieth century, dramatic advances in medicine and genetics expanded out knowledge about the genetic underpinnings of human life. The Human Genome Project, for example, expanded our knowledge about the genetic underpinnings of human life, which provided the impetus for controversy surrounding the funding of "sensitive" research. As excitement about curing diseases by genetic modification and improving the quality of life for people with debilitating, chronic diseases increased, serious and legitimate ethical issues, especially those regarding the definitions of human life, intensified. Cloning, stem cell research, abortion, and contraception each have been passionately debated in Congress. The social and ethical controversies inherent in these topics, discussed and debated not only in the halls of Congress but also on Main Street U.S.A., have been inflamed by the injection of politics into the debate. All too often, scientific evidence has been ignored, unless it supported one's particular point of view.

## SCIENCE POLICY AND SCIENCE POLITICS
## UNDER THE BUSH II ADMINISTRATION

From the beginning of the Bush II presidency, science policy seems to have been driven more by faith and ideology than by scientific facts. More so than in any other administration, President Bush and his administration have injected a conservative, religious overtone to its approach to science and to science policy. From climate warming, to how evolution is taught in schools, to AIDS policy, to an abstinence only contraception policy, this president and his administration have ignored, distorted, or disregarded the scientific facts. The administration's science policy has been characterized as one that rewards those researchers who agree with the administration and punishes those who are at odds with its policies.

In 2004, one of the most politically charged and contentious issues being discussed by the President's Council on Bioethics was stem cell research. In a brazen act of politics, the White House replaced two members (a cell biologist and ethicist) of the council whose views were at odds with the administrations. These individuals were replaced by people with more conservative, ideological leanings, thus changing the balance of the council dramatically. Researchers, reacting to this stunning action, blasted the White House on its bioethics shuffle.[11] Democrats accused the White House of playing politics.

Dr. Elizabeth Blackburn, an eminent cell biologist and proponent of embryonic stem cell research who was removed from the council, captured the sentiment of most scientists when she wrote in the *New England Journal of Medicine* that when prominent scientists must fear that descriptions of their research will be misrepresented and misused by their government to advance political ends, something is deeply wrong.[12] Remarkably, the purging of the Bioethics Council came just one week after the Union of Concerned Scientists issued their report charging the Bush II administration with a pattern of misuse of science. Not surprisingly, the Bush administration disputed these charges. Nonetheless, the evidence speaks for itself: prospective candidates have reportedly been asked to state their views on specific topics such as abortion and stem cell research, and those who differ with the administration's policies are not selected. Many have been asked whether they supported the President's policies and whether they voted for him. Concerned scientists, expressing unprecedented criticism, felt that the Bush II administration was sacrificing scientific integrity at federal agencies to further a political and ideological agenda and was doing so with impunity. For example, researchers consulting to the World Health Organization would have to agree to advocate U.S. policy or else be denied permission to consult. These restrictions went against the very elements of scientific research, including a free and open environment for discussion and inquiry.

The NIH, one of the jewels in the crown of federal agencies, funds the bulk of scientific research in the United States. Central to the approval of funding is the process of peer review. Study groups comprised of scientists and researchers conduct a detailed review of the application, evaluating each on their scientific merit. The highly competitive process is intended to be an objective evaluation of the proposal's merit and politics, philosophy, and religious doctrine are not supposed to sway the selection of the approval process. Scientists, not politicians or political appointees or advocacy groups or lobbyists, decide who gets funded.[13] Yet, in 2003, Representative Patrick J. Toomey (R-PA) sponsored an amendment to a NIH appropriations bill that would rescind funding for five NIH research grants already approved (and completed!). The proposed grants focused on HIV risk reduction among Asian prostitutes and other projects related to sexual risk taking. While his amendment was defeated, the vote was extremely close (lost by only two votes). Researchers and scientists were alarmed by the narrowness of the defeat. Clearly, what this incident showed was that "sensitive topics" would be placed under a microscope and those that appear to go against the grain of the politicians would not be funded, thus debasing the well-respected peer review process. The good news is that the scientific community reacted immediately to condemn what was going on and defended the peer review process.

The issue of political subversion and misuse of science in the Bush II administration came to a head in 2004. The Union of Concerned Scientists, a nonprofit advocacy group, issued a report critical of this administration's misuse of science. The report, which accused the Bush II administration of suppressing or simply ignoring scientific findings that did not support the administration's viewpoint, was signed by more than sixty leading scientists, including twenty Nobel laureates, calling for regulatory and legislative action to restore scientific integrity to federal policy making.[14] The report summarized twenty-one incidents that illustrated a well-established pattern of suppression and distortions of scientific findings by high-ranking Bush administration political appointees across numerous federal agencies. There was strong documentation of a wide-ranging and deliberate effort to manipulate the scientific advisory system to block or prevent the appearance of advice that might run counter to the administration's political agenda.[15]

Not surprisingly, the Bush administration disputed these charges. Nonetheless, the evidence speaks for itself: prospective candidates have reportedly been asked to state their views on specific topics such as abortion and stem cell research, and those who differ with the administration's policies are not selected. Many concerned scientists, expressing unprecedented criticism, felt that the Bush II administration was sacrificing scientific integrity at federal agencies to further a political and ideological agenda and was doing so with impunity. Since the report was made public, over 7,000 signatures have been added to the original petition.

Democrats in Congress expressed alarm about the administration running roughshod over a process that should be based on evidence rather than on opinion. Scientific appointments to advisory committees and to other public agencies should rest on objective criteria of qualifications, training, ability, and scholarship. In August 2003, at the request of Representative Henry A. Waxman, the Democratic staff of the Government Reform Committee in the U.S. House of Representatives conducted a study to assess the treatment of science and scientists by the Bush II administration. The report, *Politics and Science in the Bush Administration*, found numerous instances where the administration manipulated the scientific process and distorted or suppressed scientific findings. This action has led to misleading statements by the president, inaccurate responses to Congress, altered Web sites, suppressed agency reports, erroneous international communications, appointments to advisory panels based on political litmus tests, and the gagging of scientists.[16]

Scientific conclusions have been rejected when politically inconvenient, which sadly has served to undermine the credibility of many U.S. agencies both nationally and abroad. The CDC in particular has been the victim of religious conservative ideology. Key prevention officers have been laid off or reassigned, and a number of high-level officials have resigned in protest of "censorship and intimidation" by the Bush II administration. In addition, the agency was forced to rewrite its condom fact sheet to reflect the abstinence-obsessed administration. The edited version no longer stated that condoms are 98% to 100% effective as HIV prevention, nor did it explain their proper use. A former employee of the CDC's AIDS program summed up the mood at the CDC, remarking that there was an ideological focus being imposed from the administration that was inconsistent with the science; political ideology was being substituted for science.[17] At the Food and Drug Administration, the Director of the Office of Women's Health resigned because she believed that the administration was twisting science to stall approval of the over-the-counter emergency contraception, Plan B. (See Chapter 2.)

In light of these charges and allegations, how has the Bush II administration reacted? Not surprisingly, the White House swiftly and strongly refuted the critics who have accused the administration of systematically manipulating science to advance its political agenda. White House science advisor and Director of the Office of Science and Technology Policy, Dr. John Marburger III, speaking for the administration, took issue with the charges that the Bush II administration was manipulating the scientific process and distorting or suppressing scientific findings. He particularly found the Union of Concerned Scientists' report disappointing because it makes some sweeping generalizations about policy in this administration that are based on a random selection of incidents and issues, in his opinion. He maintained that the report distorts the administration's position, and accused the accusers of errors, distortions, and misunderstandings. With rhetoric flying back and forth, with charges and countercharges being made, there is a need to examine the record and determine objectively the extent of "science abuse" loosely defined by journalist Chris Mooney in his book, *The Republican War on Science,* as being any attempt to inappropriately undermine, alter, or otherwise interfere with the scientific process or scientific conclusions for political or ideological reasons.[18]

Both liberals and conservatives, Republicans and Democrats, are all to some extent guilty. But, under the Bush II administration, scientific integrity has been severely challenged, and in some cases, compromised. Conservative and religious zealotry went unchecked. Good science has been trampled by moral precepts. Every individual is entitled to his or her opinions, but in setting federal science policy evidence must surmount everything else. Formulating science policy in a vacuum, or worse with disregard for the evidence, denigrates the process of sound policy making. Ignoring or ostracizing scientists whose personal party affiliations may be counter to that of the majority party should have no place in setting policy. Good policy and good science must go hand-in-hand.

Nonetheless, despite the protestations of administration officials and in response to, and concern about, the politicization of science policy in the United States, a National Academy of Sciences panel took an unprecedented action in late 2004. In a report, *Science and Technology in the National Interest: Ensuring the Best Presidential and Federal Advisory Committee Science and Technology Appointments,* the panel recommended that persons nominated to serve on such committees be selected on the basis of their scientific and technical knowledge and credentials and that their voting record, political party affiliation, or position on particular policies be "off limits"; that is, an individual's political views should not be a factor of consideration. The panel took this remarkable step because of the concern that qualified candidates who held different political views were being passed over. The position taken by this panel and other concerned scientists is that the problems facing the United States and the world are increasingly complex, and the administration needs the advice of experts selected for their expertise, not their political affiliation.

The National Research Council (NRC), a leading governmental science advisory board, also weighed in with its recommendations on the subject. In early 2005, the NRC recommended that presidential nominees to science and technology advisory panels not be asked about their political and policy views. This "don't ask, don't tell" approach reinforces the common viewpoint that an individual's political views are immaterial and may not necessarily predict how the individual will react on specific policies under consideration.

In early 2005, Representative Waxman continued the themes raised in his 2003 report. He reiterated that when scientific research and the scientific method conflict with White House priorities, politics triumphs and science is distorted and suppressed.[19] Stacking the advisory committees with political ideologues defeats the purpose of the federal advisory committee system. Taking the next step in response to the growing concerns about politicization of science in the executive branch, in 2005 Representative Waxman introduced a bill entitled the Restore Scientific Integrity to Federal Research and Policymaking Act, which is designed to prohibit (1) the tampering with the conduct of federal research, (2) censoring federal scientists, and (3) disseminating false scientific information. The bill would also provide new protection for employees in the federal government who blow the whistle on political interference in science. It would bar political litmus tests and enhance transparency for scientific advisory committees. The bill further requires that the White House Science Advisor write a report to Congress each year describing the administration's efforts to safeguard and protect scientific integrity.[20] The overriding purpose of the bill is to ensure that science once again is a guide to policy, not a servant to politics. The bill has been referred to the House Government Reform Committee and the House Science Committee for review and comment.

## SEEKING A BALANCE

The alarm raised by scientists transcends all fields of science. It is not just one individual case that has captured their attention, but a widespread perception of the breach of the scientific ethic. There have been so many issues ranging from the editing of the CDC's Web site to promote abstinence and discourage the use of condoms, to the editing of the National Cancer Institute (NCI) Web site that had reported accurately that current scientific evidence did not indicate a link between induced abortion and breast cancer to reflect the administration's view to the contrary, to the altering of scientific reports by governmental agencies on issues relating to global warming and environmental and occupational health.

What one needs to guard against is letting the process of setting science policy become purely political at the expense of scientific advancement. Rather than pretending that politics and science do not coexist, a better course of action is to try to develop a transparent and accountable system to neutralize the danger of politics trampling the scientific process. Science policy and science politics must coexist in an environment that allows, even encourages, creativity. Independent and critical thinking contributes to the dynamic dialogue; muzzling those whose views are at odds with the majority party or distorting evidence to fit one's point of view is not only bad science, but also bad politics.

# —— 2 ——

# The Politics of Contraception

The political interference with the most private act of (or not) conceiving has been a reality in America for decades. Women's reproductive health has been a lightening rod for politicians of every stripe to take a stand, in some cases irrespective of the potential danger to the woman's health. Social conservatives, in particular, have long opposed government efforts to support birth control both for adults and especially for adolescents.

Throughout the long history of finding ways to control fertility, strong moral sentiments, religious beliefs, legal constraints, and gender relations often limited the provision of advice and methods of birth control. Victorian values, sexual prudishness, moral objections to birth control, and political gamesmanship often made it difficult or impossible to obtain and use safe and effective contraception. In addition to the religious and moral beliefs limiting the availability of contraception, economic barriers also prevented (and to a certain extent still prevent) many women from obtaining safe and effective methods of birth control.

Political controversies surrounding the accessibility and availability of contraception occurred at the federal, state, and local levels of government, and to some extent still do. Litigation challenging the legality of banning birth control devices, of requiring parental notification and consent for adolescents to obtain contraception, and of restricting the dispensing and distribution of these devices to specific groups of women (adolescents and minority women in particular), for example, have shaped birth control policy in the United States. The issue is hugely complex and nuanced by intense ethical and moral debates. Often, emotion trumped evidence with legislative and judicial decisions made regardless of what the research studies showed. More often than not, the available data had disturbingly little policy impact. To better understand current contraception policy, it is important to address the issue in a historical context.

## CONTRACEPTION THROUGHOUT HISTORY:
## A BRIEF OVERVIEW

Men and women have been practicing methods of contraception for thousands of years, even in societies dominated by social, political, or religious codes that worked against the availability of birth control.[1] For centuries, women and men have wanted to decide when and whether to have a child. In fact, studies have shown that out of a list of eight reasons for having sexual relations, having a baby was the least frequent motivator for most people.[2] While the link between the sex act and pregnancy wasn't scientifically proven until the nineteenth century, and the timing of ovulation in women was anyone's guess until the 1930s, it was not until 1995 that physiologists demonstrated when fertilization of the egg was most likely.[3]

Although history shows evidence of men and women's efforts to control fertility since ancient times, early contraceptive methods were ineffective at best and potentially deadly at the extreme. Centuries ago in China, for example, women drank lead and mercury to control fertility, which more often than not resulted in sterility or death. Most of the various substances that were inserted into the vagina were toxic and had the potential for both injury and discomfort. In ancient Egypt, women used a barrier of crocodile dung because it was apparently believed that the stickiness of the substance would stop the man's semen from entering the uterus, thus creating a barrier to fertilization. Ancient Egyptians also developed a tampon-like object that contained lactic acid anhydride, a chief ingredient, by the way, in modern contraceptive jellies.

Other methods that have been used by women over the centuries include a vaginal suppository of vinegar and honey that was to be inserted into the vagina. Vinegar was particularly effective because the acidity aided in killing sperm. Women also relied on folk remedies and other dubiously effective methods to prevent conception. In Europe in the Middle Ages, for example, magicians advised women to wear testicles of a weasel on their thighs or hang an amputated foot of a female weasel around their necks to prevent pregnancy.[4] Superstitious amulets of herbs and other substances were relied on as well, and probably had as much effect as crossing one's fingers and hoping for the best. Historical records indicate that many women ingested "natural contraceptives," derived from potions made from plants, native roots, and herbs. Realizing that magic and superstition were rather ineffective methods to prevent conception, many couples relied on the pessary, a device placed in the vagina to prevent the sperm from reaching the ovum. (For an excellent and informative reading of the practice of contraception over the ages, see Bernard Asbell's review.[5]) In reality, safe and effective contraception did not exist until the twentieth century.

There were many factors (social, medical, political, economic, shift in gender norms) that helped spur the birth control movement in the United States. From a historical perspective, the emerging feminist movement, the influx of immigrants, and advocacy by women's rights groups provided the impetus for the birth control movement in the early 1900s. The "mother" of this movement was Margaret Sanger, who coined the expression *birth control* and who is widely credited with spearheading the modern birth control movement in the United States and worldwide.[6] She opened the first birth control clinic in New York in 1916, and immediately, in increasing numbers, women came. The clinic represented the first attempt at a public and organized effort to provide instruction about birth control. The clinic attracted publicity, and Sanger was charged with illegal distribution of contraceptive information and jailed. She appealed her conviction through several levels of courts, and Judge Frederick Crane, writing for a unanimous New York Court of Appeals, cited an allowable exception to the anticontraception law by labeling pregnancy a disease for the sake of justifying the prevention of it.[7] But, it was not until 1937 that the American Medical Association officially recognized birth control as part of legitimate medical practice.

Margaret Sanger's crusade for reproductive freedom for women is well documented, as was her search for the "perfect contraceptive," which helped spur the development of the oral contraceptive. Ironically, not a single government dollar went into developing what could be regarded as the most revolutionary pharmaceutical invention of the century. In fact, it was Ms. Sanger's colleague Katharine McCormick's money that paid for the early seminal research.[8]

Throughout most of the twentieth century, the reproductive rights movement reflected class and racial biases. Young, low-income, and minority women, who most needed assistance in obtaining birth control, more often than not lacked access to physicians' services. At the time, there were stringent legal constraints against using, disseminating, or distributing birth control, which made it not only difficult to prescribe or provide contraceptive devices to all women who might have wanted them, but also illegal.[9] By casting birth control in a medical light, the proponents of contraception were somewhat successful in evading federal and state statutes. That is, legal victories enabled the prescription and distribution of birth control materials to prevent disease. Women who could afford a sympathetic private physician could usually obtain contraceptives. For the young, the poor, the uneducated, the options were far more limited.

While it is probably fair to say that judicial and legal restraints on birth control gradually weakened in response to social change, to some extent the fight to provide legal and safe contraception continues to this day, and the political ramifications of debate continues to polarize policy makers. This chapter focuses on the intense debate over access to and availability of contraceptives. From barrier methods to chemical methods, the evolution of contraceptive devices is inexorably intertwined with legal, ethical, and political maneuvering.

In the United States, the politicalization of safe and effective birth control for those who want it has accelerated in recent years, culminating in the debate over the availability of Plan B (the morning after pill) to adults and adolescents. The focus on this chapter shows that the availability of safe and effective contraception continues to be a pawn in an ugly political battle over a women's ability to control her fertility safely and effectively.

## Sexual Abstinence

The refraining from sexual intercourse by means of sexual abstinence has been discussed and debated since antiquity. Many religions proscribe sexual abstinence for unmarried individuals for the purpose of chastity. Abstinence before marriage was, and to some extent still is, highly valued. Abstinence advocates support this form of birth control as a way to avoid pregnancy and sexually transmitted diseases. Without sexual contact, it is virtually impossible to conceive a child after all. But, this means of birth control will not necessarily prevent a sexually transmitted disease because many of these infections, including AIDS, can also be transmitted nonsexually. There are many who adopt the line that abstinence education should be the primary focus of sex education in the United States. Indeed, the effectiveness of abstinence-only programs and virginity pledges is a hot debate topic. The evidence shows, however, that these programs are not very effective. Making sex scary or trying to control adolescent sexual behavior by instilling fear, shame, and guilt, for example, has not been very successful. Nevertheless, the politics of contraception cannot be discussed without mention of this "method."

## The Condom

The transition to a more modern era in contraception is marked by the redesign of the male condom, which had been around in various forms for hundreds of years. Over the centuries, the male condom was used as a somewhat effective method to prevent pregnancy, as well as to stop the spread of venereal disease. Casanova, it is said, favored lubricated fine linen cloth condoms. Lore has it that a "Dr. Condom" supplied King Charles II of England with animal tissue sheathes to prevent him from fathering illegitimate children and getting diseases from prostitutes. More modern versions of the male condom were made from goat bladders, animal intestines, and sheep intestines, and rubber condoms, made possible after Charles Goodyear patented the vulcanization of rubber, were mass produced in the mid-nineteenth century. Around the turn of the twentieth century, the German émigré Julius Schmidt built a multi-million dollar condom empire from his knowledge of sausage casing. As the technology improved, condoms were made from latex and polyurethane.

The growing legitimacy of the male condom was given a boost by the U.S. military during World War I. The military was fighting a losing battle against venereal disease because its abstinence program and postcoital prevention kits were not very effective against syphilis and other venereal diseases. Condom use was strongly encouraged, and American soldiers returning home from war continued to use this barrier method of contraception. By 1924, the condom was the most commonly prescribed method of birth control.[10] Yet, there were laws against contraception in the United States at the time, notably The Comstock Act of 1873, which outlawed the dissemination of contraceptive devices and information. Contraceptives were classified as obscene, and Anthony Comstock's vice squad was on the lookout for obscene (sexual) objects. Ironically, the targets of suspicion were the "street and saloon" purveyors of illicit items, not established rubber and pharmaceutical houses.[11] In fact, it was illegal to provide information on contraception in the United States well into the twentieth century, although physicians had the authority to prescribe methods for health reasons.[12]

The condom is still in wide use in the United States today and is used not only as a method of birth control but also to protect against sexually transmitted diseases (STDs) and HIV/AIDS. In addition to the male condom, a female condom, a polyurethane sheath or pouch about 17 cm (6.5 inches) in length, was recently developed. It is worn by a woman during sex and entirely lines the vagina to help to prevent pregnancy and STDs, including HIV. The female condom has been available in Europe since 1992, and it was approved in 1993 by the U.S. Food and Drug Administration (FDA).

**Vaginal Sponge and Diaphragm**

From a historical perspective, vaginal sponges were one of the most commonly used substances to block and absorb semen. The oldest reference to using sponges for contraception is from the Talmud, in which it is recommended that a sponge be soaked in vinegar.[13] Women in Constantinople supposedly shook gritty sand from sea sponges and dipped them in lemon juice before insertion into the vaginal canal. In more modern times, a contraceptive sponge was introduced and marketed in America in 1983 and quickly became one of the most popular over-the-counter barrier methods.

The diaphragm, another barrier device used over the ages, involved covering the cervix to prevent an unintended pregnancy. Whereas early versions of the diaphragm included lemon halves and oiled paper discs, the modern rubber form was invented in 1838. Margaret Sanger introduced the modern-day diaphragm into the United States in 1936; she ordered by mail a new model of a Japanese diaphragm. The package was promptly confiscated by the U.S. Customs as indecent, as defined by the Comstock law. Ms. Sanger sued and U.S. District Court judge, Grover Moscowitz, threw out the government' suit and ordered the package delivered. As a result of this case, contraceptives could now be shipped through the mail system. Women embraced the diaphragm as a means to control their fertility safely, and the reliance on this method increased significantly. By 1941, most doctors recommended the diaphragm as an effective method of contraception. As newer methods of contraception were brought to market, use of this diaphragm fell out of favor, especially during the 1960s, primarily because the oral contraceptive was viewed as being a far superior method of birth control.[14]

## The Intrauterine Device (IUD)

The history of the modern IUD is comparatively short, although a prototype dates back hundreds of years when nomadic Arabs placed pebbles into the uterus of a camel to prevent pregnancy. The pebble created a mild infection in the uterus that prevented the fertilization and implantation of the egg. In the 1920s, German gynecologist Ernst Grafenberg developed the first modern IUD from gut and silver wire. The primary problem with this method of birth control was the elevated risk of infection and injury. The tailpiece of the IUD acted as a wick conveying bacteria from the vagina upward into the uterine cavity.

The IUD was once a popular form of birth control in the United States, but with published accounts of cases of septic maternal death among women who became pregnant while using the Dalkon Shield, at the time a popular IUD device, as well as the discovery that the Dalkon Shield was associated with an increased risk of pelvic inflammatory disease, there was a sharp drop in the use of this method. The Dalkon Shield was taken off the market in 1974, and there were more than 300,000 lawsuits filed against the manufacturer, A.H. Robbins. In 1984, the manufacturer began an advertising campaign urging women to remove their IUDs.[15] The Dalkon Shield scandal, a device that was marketed despite known health and failure risks, helped kill the promise of a new and improved IUD. Gynecologists and women formed strong negative opinions about the IUD, and the conflict between costly product liability and consumer protection led to a standstill in the use and research and development of this device.[16]

In addition to the above methods of contraception that were produced and sold, none of these devices had as much impact as the Pill, a hormonal oral contraceptive that revolutionized birth control and probably helped usher in the "Sexual Revolution" of the 1960s. The Pill was nothing sort of revolutionary. It not only was far more effective than other methods, it also gave women, for the first time, unprecedented control over their fertility.[17]

## The Pill

The birth of the Pill, as it were, occurred October 15, 1951, the day Dr. Carl Djerassi's laboratory completed the first synthesis of a steroid that eventually was used for oral contraception. Djerassi and a team of steroid biochemists at Syntex laboratories in Mexico successfully synthesized the oral progestational agent norethindrone, which enabled the clinical development of oral contraceptive pills.[18] Working at the same time on an oral contraceptive was Gregory Pincus, a biologist and medical expert in reproduction who conducted trials on an oral contraceptive in Puerto Rico. The initial doses were extremely high, and significant side effects were reported (women dying of stroke and blood clots).

The first oral contraceptive was submitted for regulatory approval in 1957 as a treatment for menstrual disorders and infertility, not as a contraceptive. A few years later the same drug was submitted to the FDA for approval specifically as an oral contraceptive. On May 9, 1960, the FDA approved for clinical use the distribution of Enovid, the oral contraceptive pill manufactured by G.D. Searle and Company, the pharmaceutical company that supported Dr. Pincus's research. Of note is that this decision occurred a few years before the Supreme Court affirmed the legality of birth control for married individuals (*Griswold v. Connecticut* [1965]). Prior to that time, birth control was illegal, regardless of one's marital status.

The Pill was far from perfect, but its effectiveness, simplicity, and ease of use afforded millions of women control over reproduction. By the mid-1960s, the Pill became the leading method of contraception in the United States, helped no doubt by a FDA advisory board report that stated that there was no adequate scientific data to prove that the Pill was unsafe for human use. The Pill's status as a safe and effective contraceptive was further enhanced during the Nixon administration, when Congress established the first federally funded program to offer family planning services to poor women (Title X of the Public Health Services Act of 1970).

Continued research fine tuned the dose of estrogen and progestin in the Pill; a Pill containing only progestin was introduced in the 1970s, and a "multiphasic" Pill, in which the ratio of progestin to estrogen changes during the 21 day cycle, was introduced in the early 1980s.

## KEY LEGISLATIVE AND JUDICIAL ACTIONS

The rich and interesting history of contraception in the United States is reflected best by reviewing legislative acts and judicial rulings. Foremost among the anticontraception law is the Comstock Act of 1873, a federal law that made it illegal to send any "obscene, lewd, and/or lascivious" materials through the mail, including contraceptive devices and information. The Comstock Act not only targeted pornography as such, but also all contraceptive equipment and many educational documents, such as descriptions of contraceptive methods and other reproductive health-related materials. The act was named after its chief proponent, the anti-obscenity crusader Anthony Comstock. The law was in effect for decades, and it was not until the ban on contraceptives was declared unconstitutional by the courts in 1936 that it was overturned, although some remaining portions of the law continue to be enforced today.

From 1916, when Margaret Sanger opened the first birth control clinic, to the development of the oral contraceptive Pill, to the landmark 1965 Supreme Court ruling in *Griswold v. Connecticut*, as well as the 1972 Supreme Court ruling in *Eisenstadt v. Baird*, which struck down a Massachusetts law barring the sale of contraception to unmarried couples and gave unmarried couples the constitutional right of privacy to use birth control, contraception's rocky road to use and acceptability reflects changes in social mores and norms. The Griswold case, in particular, established a precedent that substantially changed the interpretation of the law and established a new case law regarding contraception. In this decision, the Supreme Court ruled that the Constitution protected a right to privacy. Before this ruling, existing law prohibited the use of contraceptives, regardless of marital status or age of user. Other court rulings also protected sexual privacy, notably the *Roe v. Wade* decision in 1973 in which the right to abortion was protected and *Planned Parenthood v. Casey* in 1992, which reaffirmed the right to abortion; however, this ruling also weakened the legal protections previously afforded to women and physicians by giving states the right to enact restrictions that do not create an "undue burden" for women seeking an abortion. More recently, in *Lawrence v. Texas* (2003) the court struck down a state sodomy law by upholding a broadly defined right to private, consensual, intimate adult contact, but not with a same-sex partner.

The issue of contraceptive rights became more complicated (and politically charged) in the later half of the twentieth century when minors sought to have the right to birth control information and services. Most of the concern about providing contraception to unmarried adolescents reflects the general apprehension about the rise in premarital adolescent sexual activity and pregnancy that was evident in the 1960s and 1970s.[19]

Several key Supreme Court rulings upheld principles preserving the interests of the individual teenager. The court recognized that minors have a basic constitutional right of privacy, which extends to their use of contraceptives and obtaining an abortion. Prior to these rulings, unemancipated minors had to have parental consent before a physician would treat any medical condition, pregnancy-related or otherwise, except in cases of emergency. Emancipation referred to an individual under the age of majority who is making the major decisions affecting his or her own life and no longer needs parental consent for anything, including health services. This broad definition was refined under the mature minor doctrine, which stated that a minor who is deemed sufficiently intelligent and mature and who is able to understand the nature and consequences of his/her health problem and the treatment prescribed is considered to be a "mature minor."[20] The mature minor doctrine superceded parental consent requirements. Clearly, it would be possible for a health care provider to deem an individual to be a "mature minor" to avoid involving the parent(s) in obtaining contraceptive information and services.

An increase in sexual activity among teenagers as well as an epidemic of venereal disease among sexually active minors in the 1960s led many states to remove the age limit or to lower the age at which minors could consent by themselves to medical treatment without parental consent. During the late 1960s and 1970s, numerous court rulings expanded a minor's right to obtain sex-related medical care. For example, in 1977 in *Carey v. Population Services International*, the court ruled to extend to minors the constitutionally protected right to use birth control.

Despite political actions to try to limit the provision of contraception to adolescents, by the late 1970s, a coherent body of law emerged in which two legal principles were affirmed: (1) mature minors have a constitutional right to obtain reproductive health services on their own consent, and (2) all minors have a constitutional right to have an alternative to parental involvement in implementing their decision about such health care.[21] Efforts to deny teenagers access to services to prevent or to terminate unwanted conceptions were thwarted by judicial rulings. The Supreme Court recognized that minors had a basic constitutional right of privacy that extended to their use of contraceptives, as well as to their obtaining an abortion. Access to abortion and contraception is related to the legal evolution of the right of privacy. Through the 1970s, policies and laws were very favorable to the adolescent minor; it was legal not only for teenagers of both sexes to consent to and receive sex-related health care, but also for physicians to dispense such care without fear of legal recriminations.[22]

The pre-1980 Supreme Court decisions are particularly important in that they provided a framework under which all laws and regulations must comply, as well as invalidated numerous conflicting state laws. They also are important in that they clearly upheld the right of a minor to obtain birth control services without parental consent. The political climate was such that even though there was opposition to such "liberal" rulings, the Supreme Court decisions were the law of the land.

Concomitant to the Supreme Court rulings, the legislative branch of the government also had an active and important role in legislating in the area of contraception. In the 1970s, the government assumed a more active role in providing and financing family planning programs. The passage of Title X of the Public Health Services Act of 1970, the only federal program dedicated to providing family planning services to low-income women and teenagers, led to a substantial increase in monies allocated for support of family planning service projects. Passed with broad bipartisan support in response to research showing that rates of unwanted childbearing among low-income women were more than double that for more affluent women, Title X was (and still is) a critical source of assistance for low-income women and teenagers. In addition to financing the provision of contraceptive services, Title X funds also support a wide range of reproductive health care, including pelvic and breast examinations, Pap smears, and testing and treatment for sexually transmitted diseases. To ensure that women receive services on a purely voluntary basis, clinics are required to offer clients a range of contraceptive choices on a confidential basis. There also are safeguards to ensure that women are not pressured to accept a particular contraceptive method.

The Family Planning Service and Population Research Act of 1970 also authorized funds for the support for new and better methods of birth planning, for manpower training, and for the preparation of informational materials. The emphasis was to create and expand accessibility to voluntary family planning services for adults and adolescents.

In 1978, in response to lawsuits by women across the country, Congress enacted the Pregnancy Discrimination Act. Recognizing that health benefits are an important part of an individual's job, the law required employer health insurance plans to cover pregnancy and women's related medical needs on an equal basis with other benefits. Congress also passed the Adolescent Health Services and Pregnancy Prevention and Care Act of 1978, which was the first legislative initiative to deal explicitly with issues of adolescent sexual behavior. At the time, passage of this act clearly indicated the awareness of policy makers regarding the "problem" of adolescent pregnancy and teenage sexuality. And, in 1979, the Office of Adolescent Pregnancy Programs was established in the Public Health Service to administer the Adolescent Pregnancy Prevention and Care Program mandated in the Act of 1978. This office also was charged with coordinating all programs in the Department of Health and Human Services concerned with various aspects of adolescent pregnancy.

In summary, the 1970s saw a shift in federal policy from benign neglect to one of substantial financial and government involvement in women's reproductive health. Yet, the fiscal realities of the 1980s concomitant with the election of Ronald Reagan resulted in efforts to erode the federal government's role in family planning funding and support. Sizable reductions in federal assistance to pregnant teenagers and adolescent mothers typified the administration's efforts to curtail government spending in this area.

Indeed, things began to change dramatically in the 1980s. In a direct challenge to the Supreme Court decisions, the U.S. Department of Health and Human Services issued a ruling in 1982 requiring federally funded family planning clinics to inform the parent or guardian of any patient under the age of eighteen years for whom contraceptive drugs or devices were prescribed. Dubbed the "Squeal Rule," this ruling was challenged by numerous family planning advocacy groups, and its enforcement was permanently enjoined by a federal judge. It was ruled that the notification requirement would defeat the basic purpose of Title X of the Public Health Services Act of 1970, which stipulated the funding of family planning service programs, and would contradict and subvert the intent of Congress. But, this ruling opened up a whole new debate about confidentiality and consent for health care in general and sexual health care in particular for minors.

## CONFIDENTIALITY AND CONSENT FOR MINORS

The extent to which parents should be involved in their adolescent children's sexual and reproductive health decisions is a very complicated and emotional issue. Those advocating for parental involvement mandates contend that government policies giving minors the right to consent to sexual health services without parental knowledge undermine parental authority and family values.[23] Proponents advocating for confidentiality feel that confidential access to sexual health services is essential for adolescents who are, or about to become, sexually active because some individual might avoid seeking services if they were forced to involve their parents.[24] In addition, those adolescents perhaps most in need of government-funded services might be disproportionately affected by mandatory parental involvement.

Whereas there was no federal law guaranteeing adolescents the universal right to confidential services for contraception or for STDs, many states have enacted laws that explicitly allow individuals younger than age eighteen to consent to contraceptive services, and all fifty states allow minors to consent to STD testing and treatment, and many explicitly include HIV services.[25] No state law explicitly required parental consent or notification for all minors seeking contraceptive services, but Texas and Utah have laws that prohibit the use of state funds to provide contraceptive services to minors without parental consent. On a federal level, Title X clinics have a mandate to encourage adolescents to include their parents in their contraceptive decision. Over the past thirty years, twenty-one states and the District of Columbia have explicitly allowed all minors to consent to contraceptives services, and fourteen have confirmed the right for certain categories of minors; that is, those who are parents. For those states with no laws, the decision of whether to inform parents is left to the provider, acting in the best interests of the minor.[26] Thus, minor consent laws implicitly guarantee confidentiality, but the terms of these guarantees vary considerably from state to state. Also, the extent to which parents are involved in an adolescent's sexual health decisions varies considerably. Some parents may be completely removed from issues relating to their child's decisions, while other parents have a high level of involvement.

A study assessing the potential impact of mandated parental involvement for contraception for minors found that mandated parental involvement for teenagers seeking contraceptive care and services would likely contribute to increases in rates of teenage pregnancy and would threaten the rights of adolescents to access reproductive health care, including STD testing and treatment.[27] The researchers also report that studies from the 1970s to 2001 show that few adolescents would abstain from sex in response to mandated parental involvement. It also should be reported that many studies found that the parents of a majority of adolescents using family planning clinics are aware of their children's visits.

## THE BIRTH CONTROL AT THE END OF THE CENTURY POLITICS

The Squeal Rule was just the first of many attempts to limit the availability of contraception to minors. With the emergence of the New Right (the precursor to today's religious right) and the election of Ronald Reagan, the 1980s saw the politics of contraception change radically. Challenges to the law were persistent then and continue to the present time. Over twenty years after Reagan's election, efforts to change federal law relating to access to contraception and abortion continue. Building on his "moral mandate" after his election in 2000, and empowered by the religious right, George W. Bush in 2002 announced a new federal rule governing the privacy of medical records, which would grant parents a federal right to access their minor children's medical records even when the minor lawfully consented to the services under federal or state law.[28] Even though the proposed rule defers to state law, or provider judgment, it remains to be seen whether states will alter their existing laws governing control of medical records.

## STATE MANDATES AND PRIVATE INSURANCE PLANS

Although government health insurance programs have long guaranteed coverage of most reproductive health services, private insurance plans have traditionally had no such guarantees. In the early 1990s, for example, private health insurance plans covered prescription contraceptives much less frequently than they did other prescription drugs and devices.[29] While the federal government was not taking any action to eliminate this disparity, many states enacted mandates to require contraceptive coverage. Ironically, since 1999, the federal government has required that contraceptive coverage be included in the Federal Employees Health Benefits Program, and this program has set an example for other employers in the private sector.

A study that analyzed the trends in coverage of contraception among employment-based insured managed care plans since 1993 and assessed the impact of state mandates to show trends in coverage between 1993 and 2002 found that state mandates to require contraceptive coverage made a difference.[30] Twenty-one states mandate that private sector insurers cover prescription contraceptives and related services if they cover other prescription drugs or devices. Coverage of a full range of contraceptives by private health insurance plans doing business in these states was very high compared with states with no mandates.

Of note is that in 2000, the U.S. Equal Employment Opportunity Commission found that the failure of employers to include contraceptives in prescription drug coverage constitutes sex discrimination under Title VII of the Civil Rights Act. And, in June 2001, a district court ruled that excluding prescription contraceptives from an otherwise comprehensive prescription drug plan is illegal.[31] By 2002, coverage of a full range of contraceptive methods increased substantially. Yet, insurance plans not governed by state mandates were still less likely than plans that were to cover a full range of methods. State mandates clearly make a difference.

Despite the fact that numerous states have passed contraceptive equity laws and despite the policy statement issued by the Equal Employment

Opportunities Commission in the year 2000 that stated that it is sex discrimination, in violation of Title VII of the Civil Rights Act, for employee health plans to exclude coverage for contraception when coverage is provided for other prescriptions, efforts by the executive branch and conservatives in Congress to cut contraceptive coverage and limit availability continues.

## RISE OF THE RELIGIOUS RIGHT

The rise of the religious conservatives during the Reagan administration and the substantial influence that they have in the Bush II administration is fueling the debate about contraception and when life begins. Standard medical usage defines a pregnancy as commencing with the implantation of a fertilized egg into the uterine wall. The religious right held that pregnancy begins with the fertilization of an egg, rendering most forms of contraception as possible abortifacients because, by design, they may interfere with implantation.

Numerous court challenges over the ensuing years have tried to undermine, restrict, and deny judicial rights that had been enforced. Today, forty years after the Griswold decision, there is a potent force in American politics that wishes to deny women of any age safe and effective contraception. The religious right and the social conservative's position is much more than an anti-abortion platform, although the quest to overturn the 1973 *Roe v. Wade* decision burns bright for many religious and social conservatives. The issue of when life begins and contraceptives role in preventing conception have become key political issues in the twenty-first century. Nowhere is this more clear and apparent than in the debate about "Plan B," the morning after emergency contraception. Plan B could be considered to be one of the most contentious decisions in the history of the FDA.

## PLAN B

Today, contraceptive use in the United States is virtually universal among women of reproductive age: 98% of all women who have ever had intercourse had used at least one contraceptive method.[32] Birth control is not only widely used, it is strongly supported by Americans. Yet, there is a serious and powerful movement that seeks to turn back the clock on reproductive rights by banning contraceptives in general, and the emergency contraceptive pill (Plan B) in particular. Numerous empirical studies have shown that Plan B offers a safe and effective method of backup birth control that would prevent an unwanted pregnancy. Well-designed clinical trials have been conducted to establish the efficacy of the drug and to rule out toxicity.

The drug known as Plan B is not RU-486 (mifepristone), which is a pill that induces a medical abortion and ends a pregnancy. Plan B is an emergency contraception that consists of two 0.75-mg tablets of levonorgestrel, a synthetic hormone used in birth control pills for more than thirty-five years. Basically, it is an oral contraceptive given in high doses, and it works mainly by inhibiting ovulation or by preventing sperm and egg from uniting, or else by altering the endometrium so it is less receptive to a fertilized egg. It reduces the odds of a pregnancy to 1% from 8%, but is *not* an abortifacient. To work effectively, Plan B, which can be self-administered, must be taken within 72 hours after unprotected intercourse. The drug is currently marketed with the recommendation that the two tablets be taken twelve hours apart. The reduction in risk of pregnancy after treatment is about 89%, and side effects are reported to be minor.[33] Plan B is *not* intended to be an effective method of ongoing birth control.

The first documented case of the use of emergency contraception was published in the 1960s when physicians used this method to prevent pregnancy in a survivor of a sexual assault.[34] By the 1990s, although used infrequently, emergency contraception was also used for rape victims.[35] By the end of the 1990s, emergency contraception pills were widely recognized as safe and effective methods for all women at risk of an unintended pregnancy.[36] Thousands of women in many countries have been treated successfully with this drug.

To make the drug more accessible, many medical organizations, including the American Medical Association, the American College of Obstetrics and Gynecology, and over seventy other health associations, endorsed the over-the-counter sale of Plan B. Under U.S. law, the FDA has the responsibility to approve drugs for sale once their efficacy and safety have been shown. Also, manufacturers cannot market their products for emergency use without specific labeling by the FDA.

There was no scientific doubt that Plan B is safe and effective. But, anticontraception forces formed a hard-core lobby group against Plan B. Plan B and other forms of contraception were being depicted as damaging to marriages, a license for adultery and affairs, as well as a means for teenagers to engage in promiscuous premarital sexual activity. The Director of the National Pro-Life Action Center, who is also president of the Southern Baptist Theological Seminary, is quoted as saying: "By using contraception, [couples] are not allowing the fullness of their expression of love. To frustrate the procreative potential ends up harming the relationship."[37]

Unwanted and unintended pregnancies exact a high price both emotionally and economically. Inconsistent use of contraceptives, contraceptive accidents, and sexual assault unfortunately occur, and to punish the woman by forbidding her to have an option to intervene before implantation is considered to be unnecessarily cruel by many. Plan B would enable the woman to have a medically safe option to prevent a potential pregnancy that might then be terminated by abortion. It has been estimated that emergency contraception would prevent one half of all unintended pregnancies and another one half that would have ended in abortion.[38]

Plan B has been available by prescription in the United States since 1999. Barr Pharmaceuticals, the manufacturer, applied to the FDA in 2003 to make the drug available over the counter. Based on the empirical evidence, FDA committees and staff approved the request by a vote of 23-4, but despite this vote and despite the recommendation of two expert advisory panels recommending that Plan B be sold over the counter, the FDA, in an unprecedented move, ruled against its own scientific advisory committee's recommendation. An explanation for this unusual ruling (it is most uncommon for the agency to go against the recommendations of its own reviewers and expert panels when making a decision) focused on the fear that young teenagers might not understand the instructions. Also, the FDA objected to having a drug available over the counter for some and by prescription only for others. In the United States, drugs are usually available either over the counter or are prescription only.

Barr Pharmaceuticals submitted a revised proposal to make the drug available over the counter for women aged sixteen years and older, and those younger than age sixteen would have to have a prescription.[39] The FDA delayed making a decision and called for sixty days of public comment. Yet, no action was taken by the FDA, and this lack of action was widely criticized as being politically motivated. Two senior FDA officials resigned in protest, including the Assistant Commissioner for Women's Health. In a letter to her colleagues, and reported in the journal *BMJ*, Dr. Susan Wood wrote: "I can no longer serve ... when scientific and clinical evidence, fully evaluated and recommended for approval by professional staff here, has been overruled."[40] An online editorial in the *New England Journal of Medicine* said: "This decision—or non-decision—deserves serious scrutiny, since it appears to reflect political meddling in the drug approval process."[41]

The egregious action by the FDA prompted many in Congress to investigate the FDA's actions. The consensus is that the FDA had abandoned science and was bowing to political pressure from conservatives who oppose abortion and confuse emergency contraception with abortion. The overwhelming consensus among scientists was that objectivity was abandoned and ideology and politics biased the FDA's decision. The FDA's decision has been described as being the antithesis of evidence-based medicine.[42] Ironically, in February 1997, the FDA issued an official notice in the *Federal Register* declaring common regimens of emergency contraception to be safe and effective.[43] By 2004, the political climate had clearly changed.

Plan B become the center of an ideologically divided America, and the losers, women including rape victims, are those who are denied a safe and effective means to prevent an unintended pregnancy and the need for an abortion. In no other FDA case has there been such meddling and influence peddling. Congress, for example, has not gotten involved in the review of antihypertensive medications or drugs to control diabetes. Yet, when the deliberations touch on issues where the public holds divergent views, such as issues relating to sexuality and contraception and reproduction, public policy decisions often have caved in to political pressure. Injecting politics into the scientific process is not in anyone's best interest. Religious ideology and partisan politics, when introduced into the decision-making process regarding a public health issue, is inappropriate and sets a poor precedent for the future. To diminish the process that was based on scientific evidence from well-designed clinical trials is to undermine the essence of the FDA drug approval process.

The FDA's action is inconsistent with prevailing U.S. law, specifically the Durham-Humphrey Drug Amendment Act, which stipulates that the default option for drugs is over the counter unless they are dangerous, addictive, or so complex to use that a learned intermediary is required.[44] Plan B is none of the above, regardless of the age of the woman. Also, there is no evidence that shows that access to emergency contraception increases unprotected sex among adolescents.[45] And, even if it did, the issue of personal behavior is not the jurisdiction of the FDA! Minors already have access to spermicides and condoms over the counter, which further mutes the arguments against providing emergency contraception over the counter to adolescents.

## SCIENCE, RELIGION, AND POLITICS COLLIDE

The FDA "hot potato" spilled over to those who would dispense the pills. At least twenty-three states have passed laws or are considering measures that would grant pharmacists the right to refuse to fill the morning after pill, other states are thinking of requiring pharmacists to dispense the pills without delay, some states are considering making the pills more accessible by requiring hospitals to offer Plan B to rape victims, and other states want to allow pharmacists to sell them without a prescription.[46] Some pharmacists have said that they have no desire to ban the morning after pill, they just should not have to fill prescriptions for it, as long as the pharmacy puts in place a system to ensure that patients have access to legally prescribed therapy (there or at a nearby pharmacy). In Missouri, for example, 70% of the 920 pharmacies do not stock Plan B. The Wal-Mart chain of pharmacies had a long-standing policy of not carrying emergency contraception. Yet, when the public was polled, 78% said that pharmacists who personally oppose birth control for religious reasons should not be able to refuse to sell birth control pills to women who have a prescription for them.[47] Pharmacists are regulated by state laws and can face disciplinary action from licensing boards. One Wisconsin pharmacist who refused to fill a college student's prescription or transfer it elsewhere had his license limited by the state's Pharmacy Examining Board.

Some states decided to fight back. Illinois Governor Rod Blagojevich, for example, said that he would find a way to make Plan B available without a prescription if the FDA did not approve over-the-counter sales of the drug. On August 23, 2006, the FDA finally resolved one of the most contentious issues in the Agency's history. For more than two years, the FDA had stalled and blocked approval of Plan B to placate religious and social conservatives who considered the pill to be akin to abortion and would encourage unprotected sex. It was revealed that depositions from high-placed FDA officials showed that these individuals admitted that political considerations influenced their decision to reject approval of the drug.

There was a change of heart when many Congressional Democrats threatened to hold up the nomination of Dr. Andrew C. von Eschenbach as FDA Commissioner until a decision on Plan B was made. Also, there was movement to force the Agency to reveal the machinations behind the delay. The White House let it be known that it backed letting the FDA judge the Pill on its merits. That decision effectively gave the FDA the green light to approve the drug. Those older than age eighteen years will not need a prescription for Plan B, while those eighteen and younger will, because that is the age that pharmacies and other retailers already use for other restricted products. Because of this dual status, Plan B will be sold behind the counter and will be available at health clinics as well.

Denying access to emergency contraception seemed odd. Plan B would protect against an unplanned or unwanted pregnancy before conception occurred. Those who are against emergency contraception are also opposed to abortion, yet denying women the means to prevent the need to even consider an abortion seems counterproductive, even cruel. Birth control in the United States is not only widely used, but it is strongly supported by the overwhelming majority of Americans. The controversy over Plan B highlights how issues can get hijacked by the political process and undermine decades of judicial rulings and legislative acts. Despite the significant body of research showing the safety, efficacy, and cost-effectiveness of contraception in general and Plan B in particular; despite the empirical evidence showing that over-the-counter access to emergency contraception improves women's lives and health by preventing unintended or unwanted pregnancies; and despite the fact that it is safer to take Plan B, for example, than to have an abortion or to carry the pregnancy to term, the access to and availability of emergency contraception was being severely limited by those whose personal beliefs were contrary to the dissemination of this particular drug. The FDA's shameful stalling and its disregard for the law and its own principles only serves to illustrate what can occur when science is trumped by politics. Caving in to ideology rather than evidence, the FDA's handling of Plan B has tarnished its image and compromised its reputation as an objective scientific agency.

## SUMMARY

Plan B is just one contraceptive issue being debated in the United States. Efforts to chip away at the gains made in reproductive freedom are already beginning to have a negative effect. Of note is the striking decline in contraception use over the last decade, particularly among poor women, making them more likely to get pregnant unintentionally. Among sexually active women who were not trying to get pregnant, the percentage of those not using contraception increased to 11% from 7% from 1994 to 2001. The rise was more

striking among women living below the poverty line: 14% were not using contraception in 2001 compared with 8% in 1994.[48] The rate of unintended pregnancies, which had declined 18% from the early 1980s to the mid-1990s, has
leveled off since the mid-1990s. One explanation is the reductions in federal-
and state-financed family planning programs.

Unintended pregnancy continues to be a major problem in the United States,
and it cuts across racial, ethnic, socioeconomic, and demographic lines. Every
year, it is estimated that three million pregnancies, or half of all pregnancies in
the United States, are unintended. In any given year, eighty-five of one
hundred sexually active women not using a contraceptive become pregnant. By
contrast, among women who rely on contraception (in this case, the Pill) only
eight of one hundred become pregnant. Hence, about half of all unintended
pregnancies occur among the small proportion of women at risk of such
pregnancy who do not use birth control. Unintended pregnancies have ramifications for the individual as well as for society. For many women, an unintended
pregnancy can be a difficult, life-altering experience. The economic cost is
significant. Without publicly funded family planning, Medicaid expenditures
for maternal and newborn care would increase by $1.2 billion each year.[49]
Every public dollar invested in family planning saves three dollars in Medicaid
costs for pregnancy-related health care and medical care for newborns.

Until recently, expanding access to family planning services has been a
major aim of the federal and state governments. Federal support, through the
Medicaid program and through Title X funding, has helped women avoid an
unintended pregnancy. It is estimated that in absence of publicly funded contraceptive services, the number of abortions performed in the United States
would grow by 40%. If publicly funded contraceptive services were unavailable, an additional 386,000 teenagers would become pregnant each year. Of
these, 155,000 would give birth and 183,000 would have an abortion. Without
publicly funded contraceptive services, an additional 356,000 unmarried
women would give birth each year.[50]

Expanding access to contraceptives will not by itself resolve the problem of
unintended pregnancy, but clearly increasing access to contraception, as part of
a national strategy to reduce unintended pregnancy, should be considered a
worthy and important goal. Yet, we seem to be turning back the clock on gains
women have made in the area of reproductive health. The battle Margaret
Sanger waged during the first half of the twentieth century seems to be being
replayed. Of course major advances have been made since her time, but it is
clear that contraceptive policy in the twenty-first century still hangs in a delicate balance.

## — 3 —

# The Global AIDS Epidemic: Could It Have Been Prevented?

## with Sandra Demars

In the period October 1980–May 1981, 5 young men, all active homosexuals, were treated for biopsy-confirmed *Pneumocystis carinii* pneumonia at 3 different hospitals in Los Angeles, California. Two of the patients died.... Pneumocystis pneumonia in the United States is almost exclusively limited to severely immunosuppressed patients. The occurrence of pneumocystosis in these 5 previously healthy individuals without a clinically apparent underlying immunodeficiency is unusual. The fact that these patients were all homosexuals suggests an association between some aspects of a homosexual lifestyle or disease acquired through sexual contact and Pneumonocystis pneumonia in this population.[1]

The above quote, taken from a report published in 1981 by the Centers for Disease Control and Prevention (CDC), focused on an unusual presentation of illness in a small group of individuals. The presentation of illness was something new and the medical community was indeed perplexed. With hindsight, we now know that this was the beginning of something that would dramatically change things both in the United States as well as the rest of the world. In fact, the world was introduced to the reality of a new and deadly infectious disease that attacked and rapidly killed previously healthy individuals. Twenty-five years later, an estimated 40 million people have been infected with the virus that we now call human immunodeficiency virus (HIV), which we also now know leads to acquired immune deficiency syndrome (AIDS). Tragically, it is estimated that at least 25 million people worldwide have lost their lives to this horrific disease, and millions more will probably do so as well unless immediate and dramatic treatment and prevention measures are instituted. How did such a disease spread so rapidly and in such a deadly way? More importantly, to what extent has national and global politics played a role in the spread of this disease?

## WHAT IS HIV? WHAT IS AIDS?

Dr. Luc Montagnier in France and Dr. Robert Gallo in the United States first independently isolated a new retrovirus, to be known as HIV, in 1984. To put it simply, HIV is the virus that causes AIDS. HIV destroys a certain kind of blood cells (CD4+ T cells), which are crucial to the normal function of the human immune system. The loss of these cells is a powerful predictor of the development of AIDS. HIV disease becomes AIDS when one's immune system is seriously damaged, which can be detected by a test to count CD4+ T cells. Tests can show a strong connection between the amount of HIV in the blood, the decline in CD4+ T cells, and the development of AIDS. A positive test means that an individual is infected by the virus, which can be transmitted to others but *not* through casual contact. Healthy individuals have between 500 and 1,500 CD4 cells in a milliliter of blood; those with less than 200 CD4+ T cells are considered to have AIDS.

While the virus itself is not a disease per se, it progressively damages the body's immune system. There is no cure as of this writing, and once infected, one is infected for life. But, being HIV positive, or having HIV disease, is not the same thing as having AIDS, although infected individuals can indeed pass on the virus to others either through blood, semen, vaginal fluid, or even breast milk. In fact, mother-to-child transmission has turned out to be a significant mode of HIV transmission, especially in the developing world. Estimates are that 90% of the HIV-positive children worldwide were infected from their mothers, either in utero, during birth, or from breastfeeding.[2] During pregnancy, maternal blood does not typically mix with fetal blood, but once in while a slight hemorrhage can occur at which time HIV can enter fetal circulation. It is more common for HIV transmission to occur during childbirth, where mixing of maternal and fetal blood is much more likely. Other means of HIV transmission include sharing a needle with someone who is infected; an accidental needle stick; and in the early days of the disease, getting a transfusion of infected blood.

Research shows that most people infected with HIV carry the virus for years before AIDS develops. Prior to 1985, there was no reliable way to test for HIV, but in 1985, the FDA approved the first enzyme-linked immunosorbent assay (ELISA) test kit to screen for antibodies to HIV. The American Association of Blood Banks and the Red Cross began screening the country's blood supply for HIV antibodies in an effort to prevent the spread of the virus through blood. As a result, today, the risk of HIV transmission from blood is quite rare.

## WHERE DID HIV/AIDS COME FROM?

Although medical professionals in the United States first became aware of HIV/AIDS in 1981, it is impossible to know when, where, and how the disease first appeared in this country. HIV was moving within and between countries apparently for years prior to its detection, resulting in many deaths either attributed to infections of unknown causes. In 1981, there were 339 cases of AIDS in the United States, and retrospective analyses of medical records show that at least one hundred cases of AIDS went unnoticed prior to 1981.[3] However, from our current understanding of the course of the disease, we now know that the opportunistic infections that brought these individuals to medical attention typically presented possibly years after the initial HIV infection occurred.

In the early 1980s, the "African hypothesis for AIDS" began to percolate within the scientific community. The consensus among scientists is that the first AIDS case probably originated in Africa.[4] Although cases were identified as originating from as many as eight West–Central African countries, 80% of these could be traced back to Zaire (present-day Republic of Congo).[5] Residents of Zaire had known since 1975 that something unusual and deadly was spreading through local communities.[6] When CDC researchers went to Zaire to investigate these strange cases, it was almost immediately apparent to them that AIDS was indeed in Africa, and was the cause of the high fatality seen in individuals infected with the virus.

Since 1982, scientists have been trying to understand how and why Zaire came to be the primary source of the HIV/AIDS epidemic. In May 2006, a collaborative group of researchers from the United States, France, the United Kingdom, and Cameroon at last isolated the HIV virus in feces collected from a subspecies of chimpanzees native to west equatorial Africa. This discovery finally provided the evidence to support the long-standing hypothesis that HIV is actually a mutated form of the primate virus simian immunodeficiency virus that gained the ability to infect humans. It is believed that the virus was introduced into the human population either when hunters became exposed to infected blood, and/or when the virus was transmitted locally via Cameroon's Sangha River south to the Congo River and then into Kinshasa, Congo, the geographical episource of the pandemic.[7] It is thought the mutation that enabled the virus to infect humans occurred fifty to seventy-five years ago, but this might be just conjecture. The earliest known documented case of AIDS dates from 1959 based on analysis of an unidentified Kinshasa man who apparently was infected and died of the disease.[8]

## IN THE BEGINNING ... AIDS IN AMERICA

Years before the official discovery of the HIV virus, hospitals on both coasts of the United States began witnessing a frightening and unexplainable increase of rare diseases in otherwise healthy, young homosexual men. The New York University Medical Center in New York City treated two young patients in 1979 for an extremely rare form of skin cancer that was hardly ever seen in people under the age of seventy.[9] By March 1981, at least eight cases of this rare malignancy, Kaposi's Sarcoma (KS), had been documented in young gay men of New York City. Meanwhile, in California, physicians were also noting an increase in the number of cases of the rare lung infection *Pneumocystis carinii* pneumonia (PCP). At the time, most physicians in the United States had never seen a case of PCP before, primarily because most people's immune system can neutralize the causative bacteria. Even more puzzling was the fact that none of the men with PCP had any apparent reason to be immune deficient.[10]

Case reports of homosexual men presenting with strange infections were published in the medical journals. The lay press, too, began to cover stories about the strange disease. The Associated Press and the *Los Angeles Times*, for example, were the first to publish articles in response to the CDC *Morbidity Mortality Weekly Review* (*MMWR*) June 5, 1981, report. The *New York Times* published its first news story on HIV/AIDS on July 3, 1981.[11] Soon thereafter, the CDC convened a Task Force on Kaposi's Sarcoma and Opportunistic Infections (OIs) to try to figure out the etiology of these diseases and to identify those who might be at greatest risk for developing these cancers and infections. There was urgency in trying to figure out the cause of these diseases, because the case fatality death rate among those infected was very high—40% of those infected died. In 1982, the CDC formally established the term AIDS and declared the new disease an epidemic. Also in 1982, the first Congressional hearings were held on HIV/AIDS.[12]

Most physicians knew by the end of 1981 that these opportunistic infections, previously typical only in immunosuppressed patients, had to be linked to something new and different. These otherwise unexplainable occurrences of certain illnesses were initially termed "gay cancer," because the overwhelming majority of those stricken with these diseases were gay men, but were soon renamed GRID, for Gay Related Immune Deficiency.[13] Almost all of those affected were urban homosexual men; no cases at the time had been reported from outside the homosexual community. The belief was that an infectious agent that was sexually transmitted between gay men caused the disease, and that HIV/AIDS could only affect this particular subgroup of society.

Soon, however, individuals outside of the gay community began presenting with similar types of infections. It became clear that a new hypothesis was needed to explain the disease pattern in nonhomosexual men. The first cases of PCP in injecting heroin drug users were documented in December 1981. Reports of ten cases of hemophiliacs with AIDS were publicized in 1982, and by 1985 AIDS had been noted in at least seventy individuals that had received blood transfusions.[14] Arthur Ashe, the champion tennis player, was infected as a result of blood transfusions and eventually died of AIDS. Like Arthur Ashe, an American teenager, Ryan White, was diagnosed with AIDS. A hemophiliac, Ryan too had received frequent transfusions of blood clotting proteins purified from human blood products. Recall that in 1984, there was no reliable means to test blood for HIV. Once it became known that Ryan had AIDS, he was barred from returning to school. Although members of his community were scared of interactions with Ryan, they did not blame him; Ryan was considered an "innocent victim," implying that there are "guilty victims"; that is, homosexuals and intravenous drug users, individuals who could be "blamed" for contracting AIDS because of their "immoral" life style.[15]

That hemophiliacs and recipients of blood transfusions also were contracting the disease seemed to indicate that the infectious agent was most likely transmitted via blood. Data obtained in 1985 (prior to the availability of HIV testing) showed that 90% of individuals transfused with HIV-infected blood became infected with the virus.[16] The CDC estimated that in the United States in the early years of the epidemic, it is estimated that thousands of individuals contracted transfusion-associated AIDS as a result of untested HIV-infected blood.[17] Clearly, the illness extended beyond people sharing infected needles to inject drugs and engaging in unprotected anal sex.

Another population group, Haitians, appeared also to be at high risk for contracting HIV/AIDS. Probably because of fear and ignorance, in July 1982, being "Haitian" was officially included as a risk factor for AIDS, thus stigmatizing the Haitian American community. The CDC was accused of racism, and Haiti's tourism industry (and, therefore, the majority of Haiti's economy) significantly suffered.[18] It took three long years before the CDC would remove "Haitian" as an AIDS risk factor, following the accumulation of evidence that Haitian transmission could be traced back to both heterosexual sex and exposure to contaminated needles.

In the early 1980s, when the disease was still in its infancy, people began to talk about the 4-H Club: homosexuals, hemophiliacs, injecting heroin addicts, and Haitians, who were at greatest risk of developing AIDS. But, when AIDS began to occur in women and children, many people thought, albeit incorrectly, that AIDS could be transmitted by casual contact. The fear and anxiety this disease engendered caused many to take protective action. In New York City, taxi cab drivers wouldn't pick up anyone who looked sick, people didn't want to share the bathroom with people with AIDS, and even some hospitals put up signs on an AIDS patient's door reading "Warning. Do Not Enter."[19] Also in New York, it was reported that landlords evicted individuals with AIDS from their dwellings and the Social Security Administration went so far as to interview patients by phone rather than face to face. Some San Francisco bus drivers decided to wear masks, and the San Francisco Police Department equipped patrol officers with masks and gloves to use in case they are faced with "a suspected AIDS patient."[20] A poll taken in 1985 found that 72% of Americans favored mandatory testing for the disease, 51% favored quarantine of those infected, and 15% of Americans favored tattoos for people infected with HIV.[21] Clearly, the public was confused and scared, and the scientific community was still trying to figure out the etiology of the disease and what preventive measures could be introduced to stop its spread.

Fear surrounds most infectious diseases, but AIDS was so exceptionally terrifying because once a person started to show signs of illness, they typically did not survive for much more than a year. As a result of the discovery of AIDS cases in women, children, and other cohorts not considered to be at high risk for this disease, experts modified their disease theories and concluded that personal behaviors were not simply exacerbating a previously seen pathogen, but that an entirely new virus must have emerged. With limited information available at the time, the CDC referred to AIDS in very broad and vague terms. So much more needed to be understood about the etiology of the disease, its transmission, prevention, and cure.

By the mid- to late 1980s, the AIDS epicenters were San Francisco and New York City although San Francisco had the distinction of having the nation's highest incidence of AIDS until 1994.[22] In the early stages of the epidemic, the number of cases doubled annually. In January 1983, 1,501 individuals had been diagnosed with AIDS, but by the end of the decade, there were more than 100,000 AIDS cases, and more than 58,000 deaths. By 1992, the number of AIDS cases soared to over 200,000, and estimates indicated that at least one million were infected with HIV.[23] The rapid spread of the disease was breathtaking. By 1994, AIDS had become the leading cause of death in the United States among twenty-five- to forty-four-year-olds.

Throughout the 1980s, AIDS was primarily a bicoastal (California, New York, New Jersey, and Florida), "liberal" problem, but by the mid-1990s cases were increasing in other parts of the United States, especially the south. By 2004, the states with the most serious AIDS burden also included Louisiana, Mississippi, Georgia, Maryland, and Delaware. The northern Midwestern section of the country had the fewest reported cases.[24] The current epicenter of the U.S. epidemic is the nation's capital, Washington DC, where one in seven African American males are infected with HIV. It also has the highest rate of AIDS cases in the country—a staggering 170 cases per 100,000.[25]

During the 1980s, there was a shift in who was getting infected. For example, in January 1982, homosexuals represented 96% of AIDS cases, while intravenous (IV) drug users represented 3%, but in just twenty months, the proportion changed: 71% were homosexuals, and 17% were IV drug users.[26] Also, the disease was more prevalent among racial minority groups who now account for almost three-quarters of new AIDS cases. In 2003, over 50% of the new HIV diagnoses and 62% of children born to HIV-infected mothers were African American.[27] In fact, minority women now are the fastest growing group to be affected by AIDS. Between 1985 and 2003, the percentage of women infected in the United States more than tripled, from 8% to 27% of the total HIV-positive population. An astonishing 72% of all new female HIV cases are African American, and AIDS is now one of the top three causes of death for African American women aged thirty-five to forty-four years old.[28] Heterosexual sex accounts for most new HIV cases, with the remainder resulting from injecting drug use. Low-income women, in particular, were more likely to be infected by a husband or steady partner than by a casual sexual partner (see Table 3.1).

**Table 3.1**
**Estimated Adult and Adolescent Females Living with AIDS by Race/Ethnicity and Exposure Category, 2003**

| Race/ethnicity | Exposure category | | |
|---|---|---|---|
| | Injection drug use | Heterosexual contact | Other |
| White, not Hispanic | 7,147 | 10,313 | 529 |
| Black, not Hispanic | 18,164 | 36,791 | 1,474 |
| Hispanic | 5,802 | 11,561 | 416 |
| Asian/Pacific Islander | 102 | 491 | 51 |

*Source:* Centers for Disease Control and Prevention. *HIV/AIDS Surveillance Report.* 2004. Vol. 16.

The biology of race does not make anyone more or less at risk for HIV infection, rather poverty and lifestyle are most likely the reason that minorities are disproportionately affected. The effect of AIDS on the African American community, however, isn't going unnoticed: 39% of African Americans currently see HIV/AIDS as the nation's top health problem. A shocking 63% of African American individuals personally know someone who is either living with or has died from HIV/AIDS.[29] To illustrate this point better, Table 3.2 shows estimated HIV and AIDS diagnoses by race/ethnicity and by year. Table 3.3 shows estimated adult and adolescent males living with AIDS by race/ethnicity

**Table 3.2**
**Estimated HIV and AIDS Diagnoses by Race/Ethnicity and Year**

| Race/ethnicity | Year of diagnosis | | | |
|---|---|---|---|---|
| | 2001 | 2002 | 2003 | 2004 |
| | Estimated HIV diagnoses | | | |
| White, not Hispanic | 11,242 | 11,352 | 11,097 | 11,806 |
| Black, not Hispanic | 21,556 | 20,237 | 19,310 | 19,206 |
| Hispanic | 7,714 | 6,964 | 7,078 | 6,970 |
| Asian/Pacific Islander | 279 | 319 | 367 | 394 |
| | Estimated AIDS diagnoses | | | |
| White, not Hispanic | 11,052 | 11,604 | 11,657 | 12,013 |
| Black, not Hispanic | 19,473 | 19,934 | 20,685 | 20,965 |
| Hispanic | 7,974 | 7,907 | 8,632 | 8,672 |
| Asian/Pacific Islander | 381 | 440 | 478 | 488 |

*Source:* Centers for Disease Control and Prevention. *HIV/AIDS Surveillance Report.* 2004. Vol. 16.

Table 3.3
**Estimated Adult and Adolescent Males Living with AIDS by Race/Ethnicity and
Exposure Category, 2003**

| | Exposure category | | | |
|---|---|---|---|---|
| Race/ethnicity | Male-to-male sexual contact | Injection drug use | Male-to-male and drug use | Heterosexual contact |
| White, not Hispanic | 34,797 | 13,137 | 11,366 | 5,291 |
| Black, not Hispanic | 52,120 | 34,797 | 9,174 | 21,565 |
| Hispanic | 33,717 | 18,472 | 4,361 | 8,204 |
| Asian/Pacific Islander | 2,445 | 314 | 162 | 387 |

*Source:* Centers for Disease Control and Prevention. *HIV/AIDS Surveillance Report.* 2004. Vol. 16.

and by year. In both of these tables, it can be seen that African Americans have a much higher rate of both HIV and AIDS than any other race/ethnic group.

Today, twenty-five years after the AIDS virus was discovered, it is estimated that there are approximately one million Americans living with HIV/AIDS. It is also estimated that this deadly disease has killed over a half a million Americans—almost ten times the number killed in the Vietnam War.[30]

The spread of HIV/AIDS within the United States and around the world was helped by collective denial, silence, and ignorance. The late Jonathan Mann, AIDS researcher and champion of human rights who was the Director of the United Nation's AIDS program, summarized the situation succinctly:

The dominant feature of [the early years] was silence, for the human immunodeficiency virus (HIV) was unknown and transmission was not accompanied by signs or symptoms salient enough to be noticed. While rare, sporadic case reports of AIDS and sero-archaeological studies have documented human infections with HIV prior to 1970, available data suggest that the current pandemic started in the mid- to late 1970s. By 1980, HIV had spread to at least five continents (North America, South America, Europe, Africa and Australia). During this period of silence, spread was unchecked by awareness or any preventive action and approximately 100,000–300,000 persons may have been infected.[31]

## THE POLITICS OF AIDS IN THE UNITED STATES IN THE 1980s

Initially, a diagnosis of AIDS was literally a death sentence. Although it took years from time of infection to the development of full blown AIDS, survival time following an AIDS diagnosis was a mere one and a half years.[32] For many reasons, however, finding a cure for this disease was not a top priority. For the first years of the epidemic, President Reagan never once publicly mentioned AIDS. By the time he did in 1987, 12,000 Americans had lost their lives to the disease. Reagan urged the public not to panic because AIDS was primarily confined to gay men and IV drug users. He did not sympathize with the victims or acknowledge the government's delayed and inadequate response. His focus was to promote abstinence-only education and to bar HIV-positive visitors from entering the country.[33]

The conservative Reagan government was so opposed to the gay lifestyle and sexual practices that they had no idea how to officially respond to a disease that predominantly affected the homosexual community and injecting drug users. In the first term of his presidency, when a reporter asked for a reaction about the CDC's announcement that officially declared AIDS as an epidemic, Press Secretary Larry Speakes uneasily tried to avoid the question by replying "What's AIDS?" and insisting, "I don't know anything about it."[34] Reagan advisor Pat Buchanan, however, had no problem speaking his mind when he declared in an editorial in 1983: "The poor homosexuals—they have declared war against nature, and now nature is exacting an awful retribution."[35]

Reagan, paralyzed in silence and inaction, grossly underestimated AIDS. Each year between 1982 and 1986, the amount of money that the Reagan Administration requested for combating AIDS was less than half of the amount that Congress actually appropriated (which many would claim was not enough in the first place).[36] Many prominent scientists at the time frustratingly spoke of the federal government continuously rejecting their pleas for grants and funding to study the epidemic. In 1986, the National Academy of Sciences came out with harsh criticism of the inadequate response to the AIDS crisis by the U.S. government and called for more funding to try to find a cure. The NIH would, however, take another two years before establishing an Office of AIDS Research. By that time 40,000 people in the United States had died of AIDS.

To his credit, Dr. C. Everett Koop, the U.S. Surgeon General from 1982 to 1989, wrote a very accurate, comprehensive, and frank AIDS pamphlet, and indeed, refused to bow to the strong resistance to keeping the very blunt sex and condom talk in the brochure. Dr. Koop was praised by many public health experts for breaking his previous silence and for providing the public with the factual information.[37] "Understanding AIDS" was the first public health alert aimed at reaching the entire population.

While the executive branch chose to ignore the situation, the judicial branch was quite active. In 1986, the Justice Department ruled that anyone with or suspected as having HIV could be legally be fired from their job. That same year, twenty states introduced bills that would prevent individuals infected with AIDS from holding any job that involved food handling. Transmitting the virus also became a crime, and mandatory testing of prostitutes was initiated. In 1987, it became illegal for any HIV-positive individual to visit or immigrate to the United States. Clearly, the fear of this disease was a driving force in the formulation of laws and legislation.

The public, on the other hand, needed leadership, guidance, and frank honesty about the realities of the disease. Myths and ignorance about the disease

were abundant. When President Reagan was asked about sending kids to
school with HIV-positive children, he didn't want to reassure the public that
casual contact wasn't a threat even though the experts all agreed that there was
no evidence that AIDS could be spread from casual contact, neither in the
street nor in the classroom.

## THE PRIVATE SECTOR TAKES THE LEAD ON AIDS

While the government preferred to ignore the growing crisis, those living
with HIV/AIDS needed both support as well as medications to not only to deal
with the psychological aspects of the disease, but also to stop the spread of the
virus by killing whatever bacteria, virus, parasite, or fungus was causing their
opportunistic infections.

Six men recognized the need for emotional support and founded the first
AIDS support organization, Gay Men's Health Crisis (GMHC) in New York
City in 1982.[38] The objective was to provide public health education, social
support, and counseling services. The debut of the group's AIDS hotline, in
the home of a GMHC volunteer, received over one hundred calls in the first
night. (The following year, by the way, the CDC established the National
AIDS Information Line.)[39]

The foresight and innovation of the GMHC also led to the creation of a
Buddy Program in which GMHC volunteers assist people living with HIV/
AIDS with their day-to-day needs. In its first year, GMHC raised $50,000 for
research and distributed 50,000 free copies of its first newsletter to doctors,
hospitals, clinics, and the Library of Congress. Across the nation, in San Francisco, another group of men formed The Kaposi's Sarcoma Research and Education Foundation (now know as the San Francisco AIDS Foundation) to
provide direct services and educate the public about the new illnesses associated with AIDS. This foundation started a food bank for people with AIDS,
held community information sessions, and distributed educational material.[40]
Most public information campaigns in these years were completely provided
by organizations such as GMHC and the San Francisco-based foundation. It is
truly amazing how fast these communities stepped in to protect and take care
of each other amid fear and hopelessness.

It took three long years for the government to appreciate the scope and
importance of these grassroot organizations, and finally in 1984, federal funds
were made available for community-based AIDS organizations. Until then,
these all-encompassing havens of support survived strictly on donations, fund-
raisers, and volunteerism. Unfortunately, three years later, the funds were
rescinded. Legislation introduced by Senator Jesse Helms in 1987, which
passed overwhelmingly, prevented the government from funding AIDS programs that "encourage or promote homosexual activity." The GMHC, the San
Francisco AIDS Foundation, and many other community AIDS organizations
designed to educate people about HIV prevention, HIV prevention, and safe

sex practices were run by the gay community for the gay community, and were restricted from receiving federal funds.

The AIDS community's extraordinary display of activist solidarity and patient empowerment was eventually responsible for spurring changes in AIDS drug development and distribution. In 1985, a group in San Francisco and another in New York City formed the first community-based drug-testing program. These grassroots research programs were unique in that they were formed by groups of gay men infected with AIDS in partnership with doctors. Both the AIDS patients and physicians felt that the federal testing program was moving too slowly. Doctors volunteered to administer experimental drugs and to keep records.[41]

## DRUG BREAKTHROUGHS

In the early years of the epidemic, there was a need to find a drug to treat opportunistic infections, especially PCP, which was the leading cause of death for over 70% of those diagnosed with AIDS. PCP, a very rare condition, could be treated with the drug pentamidine. As the epidemic spread and more pentamidine was needed, the U.S. government began searching for pharmaceutical companies to manufacture the drug. None of the companies the government initially approached were interested in devoting time and money to a medicine that would "only" help AIDS patients. Finally, right before the 1984 presidential elections, the Secretary of Health and Human Services Margaret Heckler announced that the FDA had approved an intravenous form of pentamidine to be produced by the small pharmaceutical company, LyphoMed, under an Orphan Drug license, which gave the company tax incentives and a limited monopoly on drugs for rare disorders. Unfortunately, the intravenous method of administering the drug proved to be toxic to many. Aerosolized pentamidine proved to be a far better means of treating the disease. The National Institute of Allergy and Infectious Disease (NIAID) announced that research into aerosolized pentamidine would be a "high priority." Nevertheless, *thirteen months later* no aerosol pentamidine trials had been initiated primarily because the Reagan administration failed to allocate sufficient funding.[42]

Infected individuals were so desperate to get their hands on any medication that might possibly slow their disease that underground pharmacies began popping up all around the country to help people get experimental and unapproved drugs. People turned to buyers clubs to try to purchase drugs that were still being tested in the United States, as well as tried to obtain drugs that had been approved and were being used in other countries.[43] Buyers' clubs would purchase drugs abroad, such as aerosolized pentamidine. These clubs were so well developed and extensive that they had drug companies abroad specifically manufacturing medications for them. There were so few options for AIDS patients at the time that some physicians would refer their patients to these underground buyers clubs. In fact, given the situation, the FDA informally allowed drug clubs to bypass FDA regulations. In the summer of 1988, the FDA would officially allow Americans to import unapproved drugs from abroad in small amounts for personal use only.[44] By 1991, these clubs were serving over 10,000 American patients and typically were run out of small offices turning a very small (if any) profit.

The first of the wonder drugs that have been shown to be effective against HIV/AIDS was zidovudine (azidothymidine, or AZT). AZT was the world's first nucleoside analogue, which could block HIV's replication by inhibiting the virus' reverse transcriptase enzyme. The Burroughs Wellcome Company began selling AZT under the name Retrovir in 1987 at the astronomical price of *$10,000 a year*.[45] Because $10,000 (or even the "reduced" price of $8,000 a year) was beyond the means of many AIDS patients, many communities pitched in to support treatment regimens for those in need. Thanks to emergency funding provisions, public hospitals in New York City were not forced to turn away anyone in need of AZT. Private hospitals, however, had to resort to donations and fundraisers. Anything possible was tried—patients shared medications they could no longer use, physicians bought stock in Burroughs Wellcome only to use the profits to purchase drugs for their patients, other doctors used money left to them in the wills of previous AIDS patients to support current patients. For others, the only solution was to "spend down," that is to exhaust all of one's personal assets in order to qualify for Medicaid, which, in many states, covered the cost of AZT.

In protest of the exorbitant price demanded by Burroughs Wellcome and the FDA's slow process of approving drugs, the AIDS activist group ACT UP (AIDS Coalition to Unleash Power) staged their first mass demonstration on Wall Street on March 24, 1987.[46] ACT UP, formed in 1987 by the playwright and AIDS activist Larry Kramer, would become synonymous with nonviolent protest against the apathy and neglect of the government regarding fighting the AIDS epidemic. Partially because of ACT UP's perseverance, Burroughs Wellcome's AZT price came down by 20%. In 1992, the government finally responded to the activism and protest led and organized by ACT UP to increase drug processing time, and started "accelerated approval" interim licensing to get drugs to people living with AIDS faster.

Since 1987 there has also been an additional government source for AIDS care and treatment funds for low-income people: the AIDS Drug Assistance Programs, or ADAPs. ADAPs are authorized under Title II of the Ryan White Comprehensive AIDS Resources Emergency (CARE) Act passed in 1990 to address the unmet health needs of individuals living with HIV/AIDS. Specifically, ADAPs are administered by each state, with the federal government giving each state a certain amount of funding to provide HIV/AIDS-related treatment and prescription drugs to underinsured and uninsured individuals.[47] It is left to each state's discretion to determine how much to contribute to the fund and how to spend the money. Twenty percent of HIV medications purchased in the United States today, enough to support 92,000 people, are done so with ADAP funds. But, as of June 2006, 331 residents of seven states are on ADAP waiting lists.[48] Even in America, people with AIDS die from lack of access to antiretrovirals.

AZT and other single-combination drugs only extended a patient's life by a year or two primarily because of the nature of the HIV virus. HIV mutates and eventual accumulations of enough mutations make the virus resistant to the therapeutic effects of these first single-combination medications. It was not until a second class of antiretroviral medications (ARVs) was discovered that AIDS treatments actually started showing rapid and dramatic health improvements in people living with AIDS. In 1995, the FDA approved the first protease inhibitor. Protease inhibitors are medications that attack the virus' ability to make the proteins it needs to infect other cells. The combination of both therapies, protease inhibitors and nucleoside analogues, led to unimaginable success that would be termed highly active antiretroviral therapy (HAART).[49]

HAART is actually a three-drug combination: two nucleoside analogues and one protease inhibitor.[50] In 1996, the FDA approved another class of AIDS drugs, non-nucleoside analogue reverse transcriptase inhibitors (NNRTIs). NNRTIs are not similarly shaped to nucleosides, but can inhibit HIV's replicating machinery just like nucleoside analogues. Another possible HAART treatment combination is one NNRTI with two nucleoside analogues. When multiple drugs of more than one class of therapies are used in concert, patients' improvements were remarkable. In addition, HAART is successful at keeping viral levels low in the body, which means that not as many viruses are replicating. Virus' can only mutate when they replicate, so HAART also decreases likelihood of resistance by reducing the numbers of mutations. In 2003, the most recent of class of ARVs, fusion inhibitors, was approved. That brings the tally of FDA-approved drugs currently available in the United States up to twenty-seven (one fusion inhibitor, three NNRTIs, twelve nucleoside analogues, ten protease inhibitors, and one multiclass combination drug).

Physicians worldwide have similarly described the amazement, joy, and disbelief of the "Lazarus Effect" transformations that almost all patients undergo after only a couple weeks of HAART treatment.[51] Emancipated, exhausted, close to death patients regain their color, weight, energy, and, most important of all, their cell counts in just a short time on HAART. In the first three years of the HAART era, from 1996 to 1999, the annual number of AIDS-related deaths in the United States fell by 50% and decreased another 14% by the end of 2002.[52] HAART has dramatically increased survival rates, transforming AIDS from an acute crisis to a chronic disease.[53] In the Western developed nations, current antiretroviral treatment regimens decrease AIDS-related deaths by 80% and lengthen lives by thirteen years on average.[54] However, because of cost, availability, and access, resource-poor nations have not seen the life-changing, life-saving effects of HAART. In the year 2000, 95% of the developing world lacked access to ARVs.[55] If in the United States, where the median annual income is $44,000, ARV treatment is unaffordable, medications for countries with average daily incomes of less than $1 was simply unthinkable.

## THE POLITICS OF HIV/AIDS IN THE UNITED STATES IN THE TWENTY-FIRST CENTURY

There is an old adage that says: The more things change, the more things stay the same. While there have been fantastic advances in the treatment of HIV/AIDS patients over the past two decades, and a tremendous increase in the life expectancy of those infected, the politics of this disease seems to be stuck in the 1980s. The Bush II administration's response to the epidemic was to promote abstinence-only HIV prevention programs. Even though condoms have been shown to be effective in preventing the spread of the virus, the Bush II administration decided to remove the Condom Fact Sheets from the "Programs that Work" section of the Department of Health and Human Services Web site. Programs that did not adhere to the administration's point of view have been targeted and would not receive federal funding.[56] The Bush II administration's AIDS policy was, not surprisingly, influenced by conservative religious politics. Nationally, some programs and scientists have been prevented from receiving federal funds because of the nature of their work.

Meanwhile, AIDS had become the leading cause of death for Americans aged twenty-five to forty-four, with the largest increase among minority men who have sex with men and among minority women. Forty thousand Americans are newly infected each year, and 25% of those with the disease do not even know that they are infected. Forty percent of those who find out that they are infected are tested only because they are already seriously ill. This means that the infection was not only untreated, but also undetected for years. Clearly, to reverse this situation, there was a need for a more aggressive, proactive policy to identify and treat those infected and those who might have been put at risk. Studies show that those who know their HIV/AIDS status are only half as likely to infect someone else compared with those infected who do not know it.

In a major shift of policy, in 2006, the CDC recommended that all teenagers and most adults have HIV tests as part of routine medical care. Specifically, the CDC is advocating testing at least once for everyone aged thirteen to sixty-four years and annual tests for those with high-risk behavior.[57] The tests would be voluntary and would eliminate the current policy of counseling patients extensively in advance of the test. Individuals would not need to sign a separate consent form. Oral notification and consent would be sufficient. The CDC also recommended that all pregnant women should be tested unless they refuse, and that oral consent would be acceptable. Health officials in many states welcomed these new guidelines.

This shift in policy would necessitate enacting new laws in some states. In New York, for example, a state law passed in the 1980s to protect the rights of those with HIV/AIDS makes it impossible to carry out the new federal guidelines. Dr. Thomas Frieden, the New York City Health Commissioner, has tried hard to change the state law, but has made little headway in Albany. The governor has not taken any sides, but many in the state legislature have stone-walled any effort to change the law. Prejudice, ignorance, and inaction still characterize the ability to introduce policies that would help stem the spread of the disease.

On a global scale, the Bush II administration has tried to address the realities of the epidemic. In 2003, President Bush signed a bill authorizing up to $15 billion in funding for global AIDS, tuberculosis, and malaria treatment and prevention for twelve hard-hit African nations and two Caribbean countries. But, while admirable in scope and purpose, there are strings attached to this largesse. The administration is trying to influence global HIV/AIDS policy, in particular on the global use of AIDS drugs, to conform to their politics, often at odds with the strategies of international health groups and often neglecting or ignoring the preferences of the nations in need. First, however, one needs to understand the tremendous burden this disease has inflicted on so many poor countries.

## AIDS ON A GLOBAL SCALE

There is not a region in the world untouched by AIDS. But, no region has been harder hit by this epidemic than Africa. There is no single reason as to why the HIV/AIDS epidemic is so rampant in sub-Saharan Africa.[58] Transmission is primarily a result of unprotected heterosexual contact, but poverty, social instability, high levels of sexually transmitted infections, low status of women, sexual violence, ineffective leadership, rapid urbanization and modernization, high rates of migratory labor, and decline of social services are all contributing factors to the region's epidemic.[59]

There is no question that AIDS is ravaging sub-Saharan Africa with speed and scope unseen and unimaginable by any other region of the world. While sub-Saharan Africa only contains 11% of the world's population, this region is home to 64% of all people in the world living with HIV/AIDS (26 million people), 63% of all new infections, and 74% of all AIDS-related deaths. If one had to provide an explanation for the rapid spread of AIDS in Africa, certainly ignorance, fear, and widespread unprotected heterosexual sex would come to mind. In many countries, migrant truck drivers and mine laborers have been mainly responsible for the spread of HIV.

The damage that HIV has inflicted on this region of the world will continue to be seen for generations. Twelve million children have been orphaned in sub-Saharan Africa as a result of AIDS.[60] AIDS has either stopped or reversed the life expectancy progress that had been achieved in some of the most affected countries of Swaziland, Botswana, Lesotho, Malawi, Mozambique, Zambia, and Zimbabwe. But, it is South Africa that is experiencing one of the most severe HIV epidemics in the world.

Today, South Africa holds the dubious honor of being the country with more HIV infections than any other country in the world: there are a staggering 5.5 million cases of HIV, and almost 1,000 AIDS deaths occur every day.[61] In just the past ten years, the overall country's prevalence has skyrocketed from 1% to a shocking 25%.

Politics most certainly has played a role in the proliferation of this disease in South Africa. Between 1993 and 2000, during which time there were massive political changes in the country, HIV/AIDS went unchecked. AIDS "denialism" and misinformation were rampant. President Mbeki consistently refused to acknowledge that HIV is a cause of AIDS, even after his own son died of the disease. He claimed that antiretroviral medication was harmful and unsafe. The country's former Deputy President, too, fueled the climate of misinformation by proclaiming that HIV was not easily transmitted from women to men. The high levels of new HIV infections occurring in South Africa reflect the difficulties that AIDS education and prevention campaigns have faced. The social and political climate has not proved accommodating to safe sex messages. An estimated 6 million South Africans are expected to die from AIDS-related diseases over the next ten years.[62] The average life expectancy in South Africa has dipped below age fifty.

Movement between the African continent and the European continent contributed to the introduction of HIV into the Western European population. The first European HIV/AIDS cases were clustered in individuals either of African descent or people who had spent some time in Africa. Unlike in America, 40% of these European AIDS cases with connections to Africa were women and were also young (average age: thirty-five years old).

The link between Haiti and Africa also contributed to the spread of the disease across the Atlantic Ocean. The spread of HIV from Kinshasa, Congo, to Haiti could be explained by hundreds of Haitian men that participated in the United Nations Educational, Scientific, and Cultural Organization (UNESCO) educational technician program in the Congo between 1960 and 1975. All male participants were single and returned regularly to Haiti for vacation and holidays. The rate of infection was incredibly high, and by 1992, 60% of urban Haitian hospital beds were occupied by patients infected with HIV. The urban prevalence rate was 10%.[63] From Haiti, it is presumed that the disease spread to the rest of the Caribbean and to the United States as well. As was the case in Africa, transmission throughout the Caribbean was a consequence of unprotected heterosexual contact; however, it is also thought that gay tourism from the United States may have also contributed to the spread of HIV/AIDS. Sex tourism provided an easy and ready vehicle for the spread of this deadly disease.

While the focus of the epidemic was on Africa, Haiti, and the United States, HIV/AIDS had not been reported in some of the most populous countries of the world: Russia, India, and China. In time, this situation was to change dramatically and with disastrous consequences. The AIDS epidemic today is full-blown in Russia, as well as in Eastern Europe and Central Asia.[64] Between

2003 and 2005, the number of people living with HIV increased by 25% to 1.6 million, and the number of AIDS deaths doubled to 62,000.[65] The Eastern European countries' epidemic is being driven by IV drug use within the male population aged fifteen to twenty-nine years old, but as heterosexual transmission increases, HIV prevalence among women is becoming an increasing problem as well. The Central Asian countries of Kazakhstan, Kyrgyzstan, Tajikistan, Turkmenistan, and Uzbekistan are located where the east and west drug trafficking routes meet, and thus IV drug use is driving the epidemic in these countries. In contrast, the spread of AIDS in the Czech Republic, Slovenia, and Hungary is primarily fueled by sex between men.

India is on the brink of an unimaginable epidemic without effective, rapid, and widespread interventions.[66] The spread of HIV/AIDS has been fueled by migrant laborers and long-distance truck drivers who engage in sex with multiple partners (sex workers) and who then infect their spouses. Widespread stigma and discrimination against the infected, taboos against discussing sex, the limited control of women to protect themselves against infection, and punishing poverty all contribute to the AIDS problem in India.

Because of its population size, China had the potential to increase the number of global AIDS cases by 13 million, or 33% of the current number of cases worldwide.[67] Initially, Chinese officials rarely reported HIV/AIDS cases, and they considered AIDS to be a foreign disease (only twenty-two cases were reported in China by 1988). The Chinese government's response to the global epidemic was to ban not only the import of blood products but also the import of secondhand clothing, and prohibited HIV-positive foreigners from entering the country. China's efforts, however, did not stop the virus from infecting individuals primarily because the disease had taken root in the population as a result of poor screening of blood products. Selling one's blood was a popular means of getting money for many rural Chinese. As such, it is not surprising that 80% of China's AIDS cases today are among rural residents.[68] Although thus far HIV/AIDS has been localized to a few high-risk groups, the virus now appears to be spreading, with heterosexual relations being the dominant means of transmission. The underestimation of AIDS cases is a major problem in China, but it is assumed that today China has one of the fastest growing AIDS epidemics in the world because of the sheer number of people in this country.

In Southeast Asia, Myanmar, Thailand, and Cambodia have the highest rates of HIV infections. Myanmar and Thailand both have epidemics due to a combination of IV drug use and commercial sex, whereas Cambodia's epidemic is primarily due to transmission from commercial sexual relations. The epidemic in Thailand began spreading rampantly in the late 1980s.[69] It is thought that the exponential rise in Thai infection rates between 1987 and 1989 was due to HIV spreading into the general population mainly by sex workers and injecting drug users. Unlike so many other countries, however, Thailand has been able to gain relative control of its rate of infection. Thailand had been on the front lines of the AIDS epidemic since the 1980s. Thanks to model prevention and public education programs, by the late 1990s infection rates had either leveled off or started to decline in these various sectors of society that are normally surveyed, although not before close to a million people were infected. Thailand has become a pioneer in the distribution of low-cost antiretroviral drugs, which are available to all, for less than $1 a day. At the same time, little headway has been made in easing the harsh stigma associated with AIDS. As more individuals are living longer, they are becoming outcasts in society, which poses a new challenge. What should be done with an individual with AIDS who is rejected by his or her family and who cannot find work?

Countries with large Muslim populations have managed to keep infection rates very low in comparison to the rest of the world.

In summary, over the past twenty-five years the AIDS pandemic has exploded to rank along side of the influenza pandemic of the 1920s and the bubonic plague in terms of fatalities. In the year 2005 alone, 3.1 million people lost their lives to AIDS, 4.9 million people became newly infected (700,000 of those were children under fifteen years old), and 40.3 million people were living with HIV.[70] As AIDS spreads into new societies, the face of the epidemic continues to change. Worldwide, women are more at risk for HIV infection than men. By the year 2003, women accounted for 50% of all people in the world living with HIV.[71] The greater vulnerability and risk witnessed in the female population is exacerbated by many political, cultural, and social factors, but is mostly a result of sexual violence, gender inequalities in terms of negotiating sex and condom usage, and a female's lack of financial independence. Tragically, women are even biologically more susceptible to HIV infection than men; male-to-female transmission is twice as likely to occur as female-to-male transmission. Women also bear the majority of the impact of AIDS in the sense that they are the ones that act as care takers for the sick and are more likely to experience discrimination and stigma, losing their jobs, income, and schooling as a result of the illness.

## THE RACE FOR THE CURE: GLOBAL POLITICS INTRUDES

The first Western world leader to acknowledge publicly not only the impact of AIDS on the developing world, but also the moral duty and necessity of the international community to respond with aid, was French President Jacques Chirac. Chirac, speaking at the International Conference on STD/AIDS in Africa in 1997, denounced the fact that where one lives in the world determines whether one can or cannot get medical treatment to prevent certain, untimely death. He went on to call for all nations and people to do what they can to ensure that the benefits of new treatment is extended to deprived populations, and formed the International Therapeutic Solidarity Fund (ITSF). Unfortunately, the world did not stand up to applaud, nor did they line up to donate to the ITSF. Rather, most countries reacted by either reemphasizing the impossibility of providing prescription drugs universally worldwide, or by simply continuing to ignore the vastness and gravity of the global AIDS status.

By the turn of the twenty-first century, the momentum for providing ARVs globally was still in its infancy. To most experts, putting millions of people outside of the industrialized world on ARVs just didn't seem feasible logistically or financially. The healthcare systems of most developing countries didn't have the infrastructure, the workforce, or the budget to initiate complex treatments at over $12,000 per year (the average price of a HAART regimen in 1996). Instead of looking for a solution, public officials were continuously and repetitively legitimizing their inaction with excuses. The world was paralyzed by what seemed to be too great and expensive a task—the potential to help save millions of lives. These excuses would run dry and, since then, not only have the Africans (and other members of poor developing countries) proven the West wrong by adhering to the strict treatment regimens, but they have shocked and embarrassed the West by demonstrating even *better* adherence rates than people on ARVs on the developed, modernized Western continents (90% on average vs. 70% in the United States). Slowly and painstakingly, AIDS has been begun to transform the international mindset about health, inequities, and human rights.

At the United Nations (UN) level, since 1986 the World Health Organization (WHO) has been primarily responsible for AIDS prevention and treatment.[72] However, during the 1990s, many UN agencies were simultaneously, yet separately, addressing different aspect of the AIDS pandemic. By 1996 it became necessary to coordinate their efforts and the joint UN program on HIV/AIDS, UNAIDS, was formed. From the very beginning, UNAIDS faced financial resistance from countries all over the world even though AIDS was recognized as a global threat.

The inequities in access to treatment became glaringly obvious to the world community at the XIII International AIDS Conference held in Durban, South Africa, in 2000. AIDS activists introduced the world to their AIDS crisis when thousands of South Africans demanding treatment marched through the streets of Durban in the Africa's largest AIDS march.[73] Just the previous year, 40,000 babies were born HIV positive in South Africa because GlaxoSmithKline (formed as a result of mergers between Burrough Wellcome, Glaxo Inc, and SmithKline Beecham in 1995 and 2000) was at that time charging $50 a year for AZT (at the dose necessary to prevent mother-to-child transmission), a price more than most people could afford. Meanwhile, ART treatment for people already living with HIV costs $7200 a year—four and a half times the collective annual income of all South Africans. In Western Europe and the United States, AIDS had become a manageable disease, whereas in sub-Saharan Africa HIV and AIDS are rampant, devastating communities at a pace unimaginable to developed countries.

Activists not only in South Africa but also in Thailand and Brazil were the first to demand their rights to affordable AIDS drugs.[74] In the case of Brazil, the 1988 constitution clearly outlined health as a human right, and AIDS activists protested in the streets in the early 1990s to demonstrate for access to antiretroviral drugs. The government had already been providing free treatment and chemoprophylaxis for opportunistic infections since the early 1990s. In 1996 Brazil expanded its program and became the first developing country to provide free universal antiretroviral treatment through the public health system.[75] After importing generic AZT from an Indian company, Brazil began producing it on its own. Brazil's biggest challenge, however, was standing up to the United States and its powerful pharmaceutical industry's attempts to protect profits and enforce intellectual property patents on their medications. The Brazilian government successfully resisted not only the World Bank's demand to stop AZT distribution as a condition of one of the country's loan agreements, but also America's threat to challenge the country's manufacture of AZT before the World Trade Organization (WTO).[76]

International intellectual property patents guarantee a 20-year market monopoly over new products or processes, but meanwhile Brazil's own patent law allowed for it to make generics to address national emergencies. Brazil also helped secure its right to produce generics by both publicizing its very positive, cost-effective public health results, and by rallying other developing nations to create a voting bloc in the WTO. The United States dropped its challenge with Brazil at the WTO within four months of filing.

In 2001, a WTO conference held in Doha, Qatar, ruled that countries facing a national public health emergency (e.g., the status of AIDS in *many* countries) could manufacture generic drugs for a royalty fee to the patent holder (issue compulsory licensing) or import generic drugs (parallel importing) without permission from the patent holder. Unfortunately, this trade agreement (known as the Doha Declaration) was complicated. The only way a country amid a national emergency could treat its citizens is to make the drug itself. In very poor countries, the governments do not have the means to do this. The WTO had to meet more than once since the Doha Declaration to try and resolve the country-capacity dilemma.

In the five years since the Doha Declaration, although the export ban clause has been resolved, only three countries have issued compulsory licenses (Zimbabwe, Mozambique, and Malaysia). The United States and the multinational drug companies are very adamant about patent protection, not because they're worried about competing with the generic companies in the poor sub-Saharan markets, but rather because they are worried about parallel importing of the generics into wealthy countries, thereby upsetting their markets in the West. Most countries that have considered declaring a national emergency and issuing compulsory licenses have reconsidered out of fear of the United States withholding foreign aid or issuing trade sanctions.

Although falling prices for ARVs hold great significance in changing the course of the epidemic, ARVs still aren't free, and were thus out of grasp for many of the world's poorest citizens. It was quickly becoming obvious that the global community needed to substantially increase funding for health programs in poor nations.[77] In April 2001, during the first African Summit on HIV/AIDS, TB, and Other Infectious Diseases, the UN Secretary General, Kofi

Annan, proposed the creation of an international body dedicated to fighting HIV/AIDS. The Global Fund to Fight AIDS, TB, and Malaria was established in 2002 as a public–private partnership aimed at rapidly mobilizing funds for the fight against these three diseases in impoverished countries. The Global Fund raises and disperses funds to governments, nongovernmental organizations (NGOs), and smaller community-run organizations. The costs of providing ARVs could be $10 billion annually.[78] Unfortunately, although pledge amounts reach over $7 billion, the actual amount dispersed by developed nations was not equal to their pledges; on average, only 50% of pledged funds were actually paid and distributed. Political resolve and economic intent are not in line with the realistic needs of this crisis.

Around the same time as establishment of the Global Fund, the former U.S. President Bill Clinton established the Clinton Foundation HIV/AIDS Initiative (CHAI) with the mission of further lowering ARV prices. CHAI partners with governments and drug companies to secure supplies of ARVs at the lowest prices possible. Because the price of raw chemicals for ARVs are scale dependent, CHAI business experts partnered with many buyers to guarantee the purchase of chemicals produced in large batches for less. CHAI also lowers costs by replacing middlemen and dealing directly with each step company involved in ARV product. CHAI manufacturing experts go through each manufacturing step to find every possible cost-cutting means. In addition, with guidance from CHAI, manufacturers cross-subsidized their overheads, thereby producing ARVs at very little profit.

Dropping ARV prices as much as possible, although it's a low margin business, can still be profitable (as CHAI has proved) as a very high-volume industry. Because of these saving methods, CHAI was able to negotiate agreements for large-volume purchases of the lowest possible priced ARVs by the Global Fund and the World Bank with many different generic suppliers. These prices are available to over forty-eight countries (representing 70% of those living with AIDS), and currently 400,000 people have been put on ARVs under CHAI agreements.[79] These price agreements have also made a significant impact on the rate of falling drug prices. Today, CHAI can offer a triple-therapy regimen at a cost of $140 per year.

On November 30, 2006, former President Clinton announced that two Indian pharmaceutical companies agreed to cut the prices of HIV and AIDS treatment for children, thus making the drugs more economically accessible worldwide. It would cost less than $60 a year per child, allowing an additional 100,000 HIV-positive children to receive treatment.[80] The drugs would be provided to the governments of the countries where the children live for distribution through public health and HIV/AIDS prevention programs.

The Bush II administration, too, has been involved in providing emergency funding to fight HIV/AIDS in resource-poor countries. With the announcement of the Presidential Emergency Plan for AIDS Relief (PEPFAR), President Bush committed $15 billion over five years (2003–2008) to fight the AIDS epidemic in fifteen focus countries. Within these countries, PEPFAR's goals are to provide ARV treatment for 2 million people, prevent 7 million new infections, and provide care to 10 million people infected, including orphans and vulnerable children. Nobody disputes that $15 billion is a very significant, and necessary, contribution to fighting the global pandemic, but not all of this funding is newly committed money. That is, approximately $5 billion had been previously committed in bilateral aid negotiations between the United States and other countries, and $1 billion was already committed to the Global Fund.

Critics have come out in opposition to many aspects of PEPFAR. PEPFAR is a unilateral project, and many people feel that the AIDS epidemic would be best addressed in a multilateral, coordinated fashion. Another aspect of PEPFAR that many people protest against is the condition that PEPFAR funds can only be used to purchase medications that had been approved by the FDA. Meanwhile the Global Fund, governments, NGOs, and all other organizations purchasing ARVs for poor nations buy drugs approved by the WHO prequalification process. In January 2005, critics couldn't help but sensing a "glimmer of progress" when the FDA approved South African generic producer Aspen Pharmacare to sell products to PEPFAR projects.[81] This represented the first time PEPFAR funds were used in the most cost-effective manner. Since then, the FDA has approved eight other generics.

The distribution of ARVs to resource-poor countries has been rather sluggish. In attempt to jumpstart the movement, the WHO and UNAIDS joined forces in 2003 to cosponsor the "3 by 5 Initiative," whose goal is to make universal access of HIV/AIDS prevention and treatment accessible as a human right for those in need.[82] Although the initiative fell 1.7 million short of its goal to put 3 million people on ARV treatment by 2005, it was significant in setting concrete goals and timelines. And no one can criticize or overlook the fact that the initiative provided close to 900,000 people a new chance at life—something that only a few years prior was unthinkable because of the enormity and seemingly impossibility of the task. Today, thanks to the perseverance and humanitarian efforts of Treatment Action Campaign, Medecins Sans Frontieres, the Clinton Foundation, UNAIDS, the WHO, and all the activists and governments that have stood up to patent pressures, the price of ARVs has fallen from an annual price of ~ $12,000 to less than $140 in less than a decade. Additionally, the cost of the tests to monitor AIDS patients has decreased by 80%.

The number of people on ARVs worldwide has more than tripled since 2004. However, although it is wonderful that each year more and more people gain access to life-saving medications, only 15% of all people in the developing world that need ARVs actually get them.

## SO NOW WHAT?

The search for an AIDS vaccine rallied scientists around the globe. Researchers have been searching for a vaccine since the first clinical trial in

1987. Yet, today, only 1% of the total spending on health product development is spent on the AIDS vaccine.[83] The majority of researchers exploring a vaccine are affiliated with governmental agencies; only two pharmaceutical companies are currently investigating an HIV vaccine primarily because vaccinations are not cost-beneficial for Big Pharma. In fact, the chief of AIDS research at the NIH commented recently that he doesn't think drug companies have the incentive to create a vaccination, and they will mostly likely wait until the government develops one. The Pharmaceutical Research and Manufacturers of America, however, insists that the drug companies are firmly committed to developing a vaccine.[84] President George Bush did allocate federal funds for HIV vaccine research, but is restricting awards to a small group of researchers. For this act, Bush has been strongly criticized by researchers.

The newly formed Global HIV Vaccine Enterprise, a new alliance of agencies suggested by the Gates Foundation in 2003 and endorsed by the heads of the G8 nations at their summit in 2004, is beginning to address the shortfalls of HIV vaccine research.[85] The HIV Vaccine Initiative, for the first time ever in a research endeavor, has advocated the sharing of intellectual property, specimens, and data among the international partners. In fact, these are conditions for the grant awardees. Another mandate is the continual evaluation of progress and failures to assure that only the leads with the most promise are explored. The initiative addresses all facets of vaccine development, from basic science to developing the infrastructure necessary to test the efficacy of vaccination candidates. Hopefully, this coordinated, collaborative initiative will provide the leadership, organization, and direction that vaccine research has thus lacked.

Yet, from the beginning of the epidemic, AIDS has been a controversial, politically charged issue that has made class, race, gender, socioeconomic, and geographic inequities painfully obvious. Fear, stigma, ignorance, and apathy about AIDS have increased human rights violations against people living with HIV/AIDS, and human rights violations facilitate the spread of AIDS. The UN Commission on Human Rights, after having recently declared health as a human right, began to take notice, and in 2000 and 2001 adopted two resolutions addressing HIV/AIDS that clearly stated that people all over the world living with AIDS had the right to ARV treatment.

## CHALLENGES AHEAD

Today, there fortunately has been progress made in terms of treating those who are HIV positive and those who have full-blown AIDS. But, there still remains so much to do in terms of treatment, prevention, and education. Less than ten years after the development of the "cocktail" of drugs now widely used to treat AIDS in the West, only a small percentage of those in Africa and Asia who need the drugs have access to them. The single-most important impediment is the exorbitantly high cost of the medications. Regarding prevention, until recently almost all foreign-funded AIDS programs in Africa and Asia were directed toward prevention. This prevention-only approach is not effective without treatment.[86] Most people infected with AIDS do not know their HIV status, which limits outreach and counseling and leads to the continued spread of the disease.

AIDS education must be an integral part of any country's fight against the disease. As recently as 2004, even after twenty-five years of AIDS in America, basic misconceptions about the disease still exist. Shockingly, nearly 37% of Americans still think HIV can transmitted by kissing, 22% by sharing a drinking glass, and almost 16% think that they can be infected by touching a toilet seat.[87] In other countries, especially the less developed nations, myths, disinformation, and denial still are prevalent.

Despite the lack of knowledge about the disease, Americans' sentiment is to do more to combat the disease. Two-thirds of Americans (63%) said that the U.S. government is spending too little at home to fight HIV/AIDS—up from 52% in 2004. This willingness to spend more may stem from a belief that increased spending on prevention (62%) and testing (59%) will lead to meaningful progress in slowing the epidemic. In addition, six in ten Americans agree that the United States is a global leader and has a responsibility to help fight HIV/AIDS in developing countries—up from 44% in 2002. In addition, more than half (56%) think the United States is spending too little on HIV/AIDS in developing countries—up from 31% in 2002. While there is increased support to do more, Americans seem to recognize the big challenges in confronting HIV/AIDS worldwide. Four in ten Americans (40%) think the world is losing ground on the epidemic; overwhelming majorities think most people with HIV in developing countries do not get needed medication (92%) and that most people at high risk do not have access to needed prevention services (81%). Meanwhile, as the world watches, the AIDS pandemic grows, outstripping prevention efforts and treatment programs and causing tens of thousands of deaths each year.

# — 4 —

# The Stem Cell Controversy: Navigating a Sea of Ethics, Politics, and Science

## with Ryan Cauley

Sitting in the far corner of Dr. Shahin Raffi's lab at Weill-Cornell Medical College's Institute of Regenerative Medicine is a beating heart. Not a whole heart, but a piece of living heart tissue that has been produced from human embryonic stem cells. Dr. Raffi created the cells by introducing them to a series of growth factors typically present when the fetal heart develops in the womb. The heart tissue lies in a petri dish and contracts between 60 and 70 beats per minute—normal for human cardiac tissue.

Roughly two blocks away, in New York Presbyterian Hospital's Cardiac Intensive Care Unit, lies Mr. Smith (not his real name), a recent recipient of a quadruple coronary bypass surgery. Severe heart disease runs in Mr. Smith's family, and despite trying to maintain a healthy diet, he has had three heart attacks in the past three years. Each heart attack has caused irreversible damage to his cardiac tissue, drastically increasing his risk for subsequent attacks and eventual death from heart disease. He now becomes so fatigued from simply walking across the room that he tends to sit most of the time. Having exhausted all other reasonable options, a heart transplant is his only hope of living a normal life. At any given time, about 4,000 patients are on the national heart transplant list. Of those, only half will receive a new heart. Over 450 of these patients will die waiting.

Few areas of biomedical science have aroused as much controversy as embryonic stem cell research. Since the derivation of the first human embryonic stem cells in 1998, the issue has been at the forefront of scientific, ethical, and political debates. Proponents of stem cell research emphasize the considerable therapeutic potential, including the possibility of curing a wide range of diseases. Stem cells appear to offer unprecedented opportunities for developing new medical therapies for many debilitating diseases and a new way to explore fundamental questions of biology. Stem cell research offers hope to many individuals who suffer from a wide variety of diseases for which there is no cure or effective treatment. But, Dr. Raffi would be the first to admit that his heart cells are not yet ready for implantation in humans. After all, there is a great risk of rejection in placing cardiac tissue derived from stem cells in someone's heart, but with more research, who knows what the future will hold?

Physicians, scientists, and those in business envision tremendous economic benefits of a burgeoning stem cell industry, just as individuals with incurable diseases envision the medical miracles that could possibly help them. On the other hand, opponents of stem cell research speak of the immorality of utilizing human cells. At the crux of this debate is the issue of an embryo's "personhood." With so many important and controversial sides to this debate, it would be ideal to have a rational and coherent national dialogue; however, in reality, the ethical and religious aspect of the issue is making it difficult to reach an agreement or compromise regarding stem cell research.

This chapter focuses on the stem cell debate and addresses the issue from a medical, ethical, and political perspective. How close are we to curing diseases using stem cells? What are the ethical and moral issues involved in researching these cures? What political issues have arisen over the funding of stem research, and how has this affected its progress? But first, what are stem cells anyway?

## WHAT ARE STEM CELLS?

Most cells in humans are committed to becoming a single type of cell with a very specific function within the body; that is, muscle cells and blood cells. In contrast, pluripotent stem cells are "uncommitted"; that is, able to become a number of different cell types thus providing a number of different functions. Because pluripotent stem cells give rise to almost all of the cells types of the body, they hold great promise for both research and medical care. For example, using human pluripotent stem cells may help generate cells and tissue for transplantation and also have the potential to develop into specialized cells that could be used to treat many diseases and conditions.

The fertilized human egg, otherwise known as a zygote, is a single cell capable of dividing into every other type of cell found in the body. The unique ability of the cell to become any other type of cell is called "totipotency," meaning "potentially all." As the zygote divides during early development, after three days it becomes a "morula" (essentially a bundle of 16 cells) and a "blastocyst" (a spherical bundle of roughly 60–150 cells with a space in the middle) after four or five. It is from the interior of this blastocyst, called the "inner cell mass," that most human embryonic stem cells are derived.[1] As the embryo divides, this small mass of cells begins to "differentiate" into other less potent stem cell types. Each time these cells differentiate, they can potentially become fewer different types of cells. Stem cells that can no longer become every type of cell in the human body are called "multipotent" cells, loosely translating to "potentially many" (but not all). Eventually, each of the stem cells differentiates into "committed" cells. These committed cells can sometimes still divide and produce copies of themselves, but they can never become any other type of cell.[2]

Although stem cells are present in the greatest quantities during human embryonic development, there are still some stem cells maintained in the adult human body, albeit in very small quantities. It is thought that in most tissues, these "adult stem cells" provide a source of new cells to replace those lost because of organ damage or natural cell death. These adult stem cells produce copies of themselves throughout the lifetime of the organism, providing a permanent source of repair.[3] Although these are similar in some ways to human embryonic stem cells, they differ in several key ways. Most important, adult stem cells are all "multipotent," meaning that they can only develop into a finite number of cell types. For example, stem cells derived from adult bone marrow, where blood is made, can only become blood cells, and not liver, heart, or nerve cells.[4] As such, adult stem cells may have limited potential compared with pluripotent stem cells derived from embryos or fetal tissue. Many researchers are attempting to find ways to "de-differentiate" these cells, in essence turning them back into pluripotent stem cells. While adult stem cells can be useful in certain therapies, they are not as potentially powerful as the embryonic stem cell, which can become any other type of cell in the human body.

## HISTORY OF STEM CELL RESEARCH

In the early 1900s, scientists began to postulate that all blood cells came from a type of master progenitor cell or stem cell. They theorized that it was this master cell, residing in the marrow of adult bone tissue, that provided the body with a continual source of new red and white blood cells. These cells are called hematopoietic cells (stem cells that form blood and immune cells and are responsible for the constant renewal of blood), and are considered to be of vital importance to the blood and immune systems. The white blood cells that these stem cells can produce, for example, are absolutely crucial for every human's ability to fight off infection.[5]

In 1953, almost by accident, research on stem cells began. While investigating the effects of cigarette papers and tobacco on laboratory mice, a young scientist named Leroy Stevens noticed a tumor in one of his lab mice. Strangely, this tumor seemed to be completely unrelated to the effects of the smoking trials. Located in the testicles of one of his adult male mice, the tumor was found to be a teratoma, or a mass of wrongly differentiated cells, containing bone, teeth, and hair. Dr. Stevens found that by injecting stem cells derived from the inner cell mass of embryonic mouse blastocysts into the testes of other mice, he could induce the formation of a teratoma. In a series of experiments, he proved that stem cells could both be derived from the embryo and forced to differentiate when placed in a live organism.[6] A year later, in 1954, Dr. John Enders of Harvard University began to use stem cells derived from a fetal kidney to produce poliovirus. For this work, Dr. Enders would later be awarded the Nobel Prize in Medicine.

It wasn't until the late 1960s that the first medical therapies based on the use of stem cells became available. In 1968, several children with severe immune deficiency disorder (also known as "bubble boy disorder," where no white blood cells are made) were successfully given bone marrow transplants. After the transplants, the children were found to be making new white blood cells, proving that the transplanted marrow both contained blood stem cells, and that these cells were capable of surviving and dividing in a new organism.[7]

In the 1970s and 1980s, embryonic stem cells derived from blastocysts were demonstrated to spontaneously give rise to a number of different cell types while allowing them to divide and replicate in a petri dish. Probably the most exciting discovery related to stem cell research occurred in 1996, when scientists at the Roslin Institute in Scotland announced the birth of Dolly the Sheep, the first animal cloned from adult cells. To clone Dolly from her "mother," the scientists had taken skin cells from an adult sheep, extracted the genetic information, and placed it into a fertilized sheep egg (with its genetic information already removed). This fertilized egg, now with Dolly's mother's genes, was then implanted in the womb of a surrogate sheep to be allowed to come to term. Several months later Dolly was born, and history was made.[8]

Researchers in the United States, too, were working in this nascent field. In 1998, two separate research teams led by Drs. James Thompson of the University of Wisconsin and John Gearhart of Johns Hopkins University developed the first embryonic stem cell lines. In both cases, the research was funded privately (no federal funds were used). Stem cell lines are stem cells that have been placed in a petri dish and induced to replicate, producing a permanent source of identical stem cells. Dr. Thompson and his colleagues derived their cell line from cells taken from surplus embryos donated voluntarily by couples undergoing fertility treatment at an in vitro fertilization clinic (IVF).[9] Dr. Gearhart's cell line, from early, nonliving fetuses obtained from first trimester abortions, produced cells that could be replicated indefinitely and were shown to have the potential to grow into any tissue or organ in the body, thus holding great promise for treatment and cures. Prior to this time, animal embryos were the only source of embryonic stem cells.

In response to these groundbreaking studies, in 1999 the journal *Science*, in a special cover article and editorial, declared pluripotent stem cell research to be the scientific "breakthrough" of the year.[10]

## HOW ARE STEM CELL LINES MADE?

Stem cells can come from several different sources in the human body, specifically from adult organs and tissues, embryonic tissues, and most recently from umbilical cord blood, which possesses a high concentration of stem cells. Adult stem cells are drawn from blood and bone marrow rather than from embryos. Because stem cells are present in greater quantities in adult bone marrow than in most other adult tissues, it is not surprising that marrow was one of the first places that adult stem cells were successfully harvested and used therapeutically.

Adult stem cells have been used therapeutically since the 1960s, when the first successful bone marrow transplants were performed. Yet stem cell lines are far more difficult to create and maintain when starting with adult stem cells. Adult stem cells can be made to divide and replicate in culture; however, scientists have found that they often cannot induce the cells to divide indefinitely. After a certain number of divisions, the cell lines will simply die.[11] Until quite recently, it was thought that stem cells originating from adult organs could only become cells found in the organ from which the stem cell was taken. In other words, it was thought that stem cells in liver could only make liver cells, and stem cells found in the nervous system could only make nerve cells. However, several experiments in the past couple of years found that stem cells originating from one organ can possibly still become cells of another organ type if encouraged in "the right way." For example, some researchers[12] have shown that adult liver cells could be transformed relatively easily into insulin-producing pancreas cells, but clearly more research must be conducted to explore this issue more fully.

Embryonic tissues have always been the most reliable source of stem cell lines. Stem cells called embryonic stem cells are found in great quantities in the human embryo. Pluripotent stem cell lines can be derived from early embryos before they implant in the uterus. To create embryonic stem cell lines, cells from the inner cell mass of the blastocyst are removed and cultured, but this process means that the embryo cannot implant in the uterus.

The greatest advantage of using embryonic stem cells is their "totipotency," or ability to become any type of cell. A single stem cell line from an embryo could therefore potentially cure a larger range of diseases than a single stem cell line from an adult organ (unless the adult line could be scientifically modified to be totipotent). In addition, large numbers of embryonic stem cells can be grown relatively easily in culture. By placing the cells in petri dishes with feeder cells (which help support the stem cells) and several chemical agents, embryonic stem cells will divide and flourish indefinitely. In fact, the first embryonic stem cell lines created during the late 1990s are healthy and continue to divide to this day.[13] With thousands of surplus embryos, the byproducts of IVF therapy, embryonic stem cells theoretically are readily available for research purposes.

Umbilical cord blood is a new and potentially exciting source of adult stem cells. The blood, which is now often collected from the umbilical cord after birth, is typically rich in several different types of adult stem cells (though the majority are blood stem cells). Because the collection procedure is painless and quick, it is possible that this could be a major source of stem cells in the future.

In fact, in 2003, Congress passed the Cord Blood Stem Cell Act to establish a national network to prepare, store, and distribute the cells. Just after this act was passed, NGOs such as the National Bone Marrow Donation Center and the Red Cross also began to set up national cord blood banking programs to encourage the donation of cord blood and take advantage of this rich source of cells.[14]

## STEM CELL RESEARCH AND CLONING

One goal of stem cell research is to provide cells that could be implanted in humans to repair damaged organs and tissues. The range of diseases that could be helped by this type of therapy is tremendous. However, there are many considerations that need to be taken into account when placing foreign material in any human being. First and foremost, there is the consideration of the possibility of rejection. The human body has an excellent immune system built to recognize foreign material, so when a foreign organ is transplanted into an individual, the individual's immune system will work to attack and destroy the organ. For this reason, organs must be "matched" to their recipient to minimize the chance of rejection. Using a series of complex tests, doctors can tell the likelihood of a certain individual rejecting a given organ. Of course, except in the case of identical twins, no donor is going to completely genetically match a recipient. Therefore, doctors have discovered that by using a cocktail of drugs, they can suppress or "turn off" the immune system so that the transplanted organ can survive. Because these types of immune suppression therapies can wreak havoc on an individual, leaving them more at risk of infection, they are only used when absolutely necessary.

In stem cell therapies, a foreign body, albeit a much smaller one, is being transplanted into an individual. If the stem cell line is not a complete genetic match for the recipient, there will be an immune response that will reject the foreign stem cells. It is, therefore, of utmost importance to either (1) have stem cells that will be a complete genetic match for the recipient, or (2) have a sufficient number of unique stem cell lines available so that a near-perfect match can be made. In this vein, scientists have begun to conceive of ways to produce stem cell lines that satisfy these criteria. One possibility for creating genetically identical stem cells is therapeutic cloning.

Cloning is a time-intensive and expensive process. Theoretically, only one human egg is required to create each new stem cell line. However, therapeutic cloning is actually quite a bit more difficult than this implies. Using current techniques, only 1% of eggs that have been injected with new genetic information go on to become stem cell lines. This means that for each stem cell line that is created, over one hundred eggs will be needed. Each egg will need to be donated by women willing to undergo the painful procedure of egg harvesting. While doctors are now making great strides in increasing the yield of stem cell lines from cloned eggs in mouse studies, much work is still being done to continue to improve the process.

Through the use of therapeutic cloning, it is possible to produce embryonic stem cell lines that are perfect genetic matches for patients. Reaching this goal would mean being one step closer to realizing the tremendous therapeutic potential that embryonic stem cells appear to offer for the future. The stakes are high, and the pressure to be the first to produce stem cell lines by cloning cells can lead some to take irresponsive action. The biggest scandal to date occurred in South Korea.

The South Korean scientist Dr. Hwang Woo Suk and his colleagues at Seoul National University published a paper in the acclaimed journal *Science* in 2004 claiming to have produced stem cell lines by cloning cells derived from adult patients.[15] The researchers alleged that these cell lines were genetically identical to the patients from whom they were cloned, and therefore perfect for future stem cell therapy. Scientists around the globe became ecstatic, because their goal of using genetically identical stem cells for "personalized medicine" seemed closer than ever to being realized. Dr. Hwang's apparent accomplishments were received by the medical establishment as a harbinger of future success in embryonic stem cell research. His experiments were deemed to be proof of the success of stem cell research and were used to justify increases in state and private spending. But, in December 2005, Dr. Hwang admitted to falsifying his experimental records and abruptly resigned from his university post.[16] A panel of investigators found that Dr. Hwang's laboratory had no record of ever having successfully created a genetically identical stem cell line through the use of cloning.

As this unfortunate example shows, we are still a long way off from using therapeutic cloning to cure disease.

## THE POTENTIAL OF STEM CELL RESEARCH

Millions of people suffer from a wide range of diseases, many of which are either very difficult to treat or are incurable with current medical therapies. The potential use of stem cell therapy to affect a cure, or ameliorate symptoms, is fueling research. For example, leukemia, a very difficult type of blood cancer, is being treated through cord blood therapies because research has shown that stem cells from cord blood are a viable alternative to bone marrow as a source of new blood stem cells. In children, this disease is often treated through the use of radiation or chemical therapy, followed by bone marrow transplants. Current stem cell studies have shown that using stem cells derived from umbilical cord blood is a viable alternative to bone marrow as a source of new blood stem cells. In fact, it was recently suggested that cord blood stem cells may not have to be as closely genetically matched to a recipient to avoid detection and rejection by the patient's immune system.[17] Because cancer patients often do not have relatives that would be suitable genetic matches for bone marrow donation, cord blood from unrelated donors could potentially be a lifesaving alternative.

Recent animal trials have shown partially restored eyesight in mammals with macular degeneration, the most common cause of blindness in human beings (essentially due to older age).[18] Research is focusing on isolating adult stem cells from a blind individual and reimplanting these cells in a patient's retina. If successful, this technique could revolutionize the way physicians treat blindness. Much work still needs to be done, of course, to be sure that this kind of therapy will be feasible.

Spinal cord trauma has always been one of the most difficult injuries for physicians to treat. Unlike the cells of our skin, which can divide and replace themselves when the skin is cut or damaged, nerve cells are not normally capable of regeneration. For many years it was thought that spinal cord cells would never be capable of repair, leaving little hope for people with spinal cord injuries. It wasn't until the discovery of stem cells that a means to repair spinal cord injuries was even considered. In 1999, in one of the first studies using embryonic stem cells (ES), McDonald et al.[19] demonstrated that ES cells could be used to improve the mobility of rats with spinal cord injuries. By transplanting ES cells taken from a fetal rat's spinal cord, the researchers were able to markedly improve mobility and strength in adult rats that had sustained spinal cord trauma. Interestingly, they found that the implanted cells were able to survive and differentiate into various types of functional nerve cells. Building on this finding, Wichterle et al. found that ES cells could be transformed into nerve cells by introducing them to a series of previously known chemical signals in petri dishes.[20] Once these cells were transformed, they could then be used to repair rat spinal cords, resulting in the return of even greater motor control than in the McDonald studies.

The repair of heart tissue has often been seen as a holy grail for cardiac researchers. Nearly 700,000 Americans died of heart disease in 2002, now the leading cause of death in the United States.[21] At present, it is impossible to reverse the heart damage that inevitably occurs during a myocardial infarction, the major cause of cardiac-related deaths. If heart tissue could be replaced or repaired, it would be possible to greatly reduce the catastrophic nature of this illness. As is the case with spinal cord damage, ES cells offer one of the most promising therapies for the repair of cardiac tissue. Two of the most dangerous areas of the heart to damage in a heart attack are the SA and AV nodes, otherwise known as the pacemakers of the heart. The pacemaker region sends a highly rhythmic signal that causes the rest of the heart to beat. When the pacemaker is damaged, the heart often begins to beat at a dangerously low rate. The current therapy for people with pacemaker damage is the implantation of an electronic pacemaker. As with any heart surgery, the implantation of an artificial pacemaker poses a considerable amount of risk to patients and can lead to many more cardiac complications than a natural pacemaker. If the heart's pacemaker could be repaired using ES cells, it is possible that the result would be far more stable and reliable than the current electronic therapies.

In 2004, Kehat et al. created a series of myocardial cell grafts from ES cells using a set of growth factors known to cause stem cells to become cardiac tissue.[22] These grafts were then transplanted into pigs that had sustained damage to the AV node, the second pacemaker of the heart. Once transplanted, the pigs' hearts began to beat at a much quicker and healthier rate.

In another exciting study, researchers at Weill-Cornell Medical College and Memorial Sloane-Kettering Cancer Institute found that congenital heart defects could be repaired in utero using ES cells.[23,24] Congenital heart defects can be highly lethal for newborns and are often difficult to surgically repair at birth. Amazingly, these researchers found that congenital heart defects could be partially repaired simply by injecting ES cells into the afflicted fetal mouse's mother. After being injected, the ES cells were found to secrete certain growth factors and chemical signals that caused the offspring's own heart cells to regenerate themselves.

Stem cells from umbilical cord blood could be a potential boon for tissue regeneration therapies. Umbilical cord blood is a valuable source of endothelial progenitor cells, a type of cells vital for tissue engineering. In 2005, researchers from the University of Zurich found that by placing these stem cells on bio-absorbable scaffolding, it was possible to create strips of tissue that could be molded into any form. Using this method, they were able to create patches and valves that could be used to repair damaged blood vessels and heart tissue.[25]

Among those suffering from Parkinson's disease (PD), a neurodegenerative disorder primarily characterized by the loss of nerve cells within the brain that secrete the neurotransmitter dopamine, stem cell research is viewed as a mean of alleviating a host of symptoms, including tremors, muscle rigidity, and a general slowing of physical movement. This debilitating neurodegenerative disease affects over 5.5 million Americans. Embryonic stem cells have been viewed as being useful in treating those with Parkinson's disease. Currently, there are two main types of therapy: dopamine boosting medication and deep brain stimulation. Medication, which had been the primary mode of therapy, mainly focuses on increasing the amount of dopamine in the brain. By increasing the amount of dopamine, symptoms are often, but not always, reduced considerably. Deep brain stimulation is a recently discovered surgical intervention in which a stimulator is implanted in a certain area of the brain.[26] By sending an electronic signal, the stimulator attempts to interfere with the rapid and wayward neural signals that occur in many PD patients. By interfering with these signals, it is possible to alleviate the tremors that are associated with the disease. But, both of these treatments only lead to a reduction, and not a complete elimination, of Parkinson's symptoms. In addition, as the disease progresses, these treatments become less and less effective.

The main dilemma in PD is the loss of dopamine-secreting neurons; therefore, to treat PD scientists must first be able to create these neurons from ES cells. Takagi et al.[27], of Kyoto University in Japan, were the first to do so at the end of 2004. When these newly created dopamine-secreting neurons were implanted in monkeys with symptoms of PD, tremors were significantly reduced.

Diabetes currently affects over 16 million Americans. As obesity rates sky rocket in the United States, adult onset diabetes mellitus is increasingly prevalent.[28] Diabetes can lead to a host of problems throughout a person's life, including blindness, loss of limb function, heart disease, and kidney failure. Current diabetes therapies are based on the replacement of insulin through the use of pills or an injection, depending upon how much insulin is needed. To match insulin dosage with blood glucose levels (which fluctuate throughout the day), diabetics are often required to test their glucose levels several times each day. The goal is to maintain this delicate balance of insulin and glucose to keep glucose levels as close to normal as possible. Stem cells are being considered as a means to help diabetics better regulate their insulin. In October of 2005, three scientists at the University of Wisconsin announced that they had produced synthetic beta islet cells using ES cells in rats.[29]

President Ronald Reagan's death from Alzheimer's disease triggered an outpouring of support for embryonic stem cell research. But, in contrast to PD, diabetes, and spinal injuries, Alzheimer's disease involves the loss of huge numbers and varieties of nerve cells in the brain. The complexity of the brain makes stem cells an unlikely therapy for this disease.

In summary, despite the stunning advances in stem cell research, so much more still needs to be understood before individuals could be treated on a large scale. While early research results are extremely promising, nonscientific issues have clouded the issue. Discussion and debate tend to ignore the scientific merits of stem cell use and focus on the larger and more difficult ethical and moral issues. The crux of the matter is that the extraction of human stem cells to create a stem cell line currently requires the destruction of a harvested embryo, and debate is now focused on the status of the embryo. Is it a living "human being"? Should embryos be destroyed for the sake of future advances in medical science?

## ETHICAL ISSUES

The human embryonic stem cell debate is often framed as part of a larger discussion on the ethics of this technology. The extraction of human stem cells to create a stem cell line currently requires the destruction of the harvested embryo. As a result, the question of the embryo's moral status is often considered the most controversial question in the stem cell research debate. At the center of the dialogue is the question of an embryo's "personhood." Do embryonic stem cells represent a life? That is, are the pluripotent stem cells human and have the same rights as born humans? Are pluripotent embryonic stem cells morally protected entities, or are they more like other disposable tissues gleaned from the human body?[30] The crux of the question focuses on when life begins, for which there is no easy answer.

A current method of avoiding this controversy has been to find ways to extract stem cells without harming or destroying a human embryo. It has been thought that by discovering benign harvesting techniques, stem cell research could be unhampered by the ethical and religious debates surrounding the question of the embryos personhood and human right to life.

Two new methods for producing pluripotent stem cell lines have shown promise. The use of preimplantation genetic diagnosis (PGD) for the harvesting of embryonic stem cells is a benign procedure that has been used by IVF clinics for many years to determine the genetic health of embryos before their implantation in the mother's uterus. By using this technique, IVF clinics can avoid using embryos that are predisposed to developing lethal genetic diseases such as Tay Sachs, Huntingtons, muscular dystrophy, and cystic fibrosis. Since two days after the meeting of the sperm and the egg an embryo consists of only eight cells, by using special techniques, it is possible to remove a single cell while allowing the remaining cells to develop into a human being.[31]

Alexander Meissner and Rudolf Jaenisch of the Whitehead Institute for Biomedical Research recently suggested another alternative for creating stem cell lines without causing the destruction of an embryo: alternative nuclear transfer (ANT), which is designed to create a modified cell that is incapable of fully developing into a human individual.[32] Meissner and Jaenisch believe that if the cell cannot become a human, it cannot be considered to possess personhood.

The response to both of these alternative techniques has been highly varied. After the announcement of the new methods in the Journal *Nature,* a spokesman from the U.S. Conference of Catholic Bishops stated that while the two reported techniques still raise some ethical questions, they do represent "a step in the right direction."[33] Some social conservative leaders such as Representative Roscoe G. Bartlett of Maryland, a self-described prolife advocate, believe that "except for the small minority in the pro-life community that doesn't even support IVF therapy, [these techniques] circumvent all of the ethical arguments against stem cell research."[34] Other leaders, like Dr. John Shea, medical advisor to the Campaign for Life Coalition, came out against these techniques, saying that the PGD technique does not benefit the child and thus cannot be used without the child (embryo's) consent.[35] Similarly, Tony Perkins of the Family Research Council, wrote that "it is not clear what effect [PGD] would have on the children born after having had one of their cells removed."[36] And, Richard Doerflinger, deputy director of prolife activities at the U.S. Catholic Bishops Conference, discouraged the use of either technique. PGD, he stated, "places the embryo at unreasonable risk," and ANT appears to "create an embryo for the purposes of destroying it."[37]

And the debate continues. But, what if stem cells could be produced without embryo loss? Would this then make a difference? As it happens, a small biotech company says that it has found a way to produce human embryonic stem cells without destroying an embryo.[38] Researchers at Advanced Cell Technology grew a colony of stem cells, leaving the embryo unharmed, from a single cell removed from an embryo that had only eight to ten cells. Presently, physicians routinely remove a cell from an eight-cell embryo to screen for chromosomal abnormalities prior to implantation. Hence, logic has it that deriving stem cells from this method adds no additional risk since a diagnostic screening procedure already relies on this technique.

The questions that need answering are: Would this new technique satisfy those who believe that it is unethical to remove a cell purely for stem cell research? Would this technique satisfy those who believe that life is being destroyed? For those who believe that a single cell removed from an early embryo may have the potential to produce life this new technique probably will not change their mind. For those who are proponents of stem cell research, what this newest development shows is that stem cells can be produced without destroying an embryo and does not destroy the potential for life. Dr. Robert Lanza, the senior researcher on the Advanced Cell Technology study, believes that there is no evidence that a single stem cell, once replication has begun, has the intrinsic capacity to generate a complete organism when extracted during the blastomere stage (consisting of eight cells).[39] In addition, unless proven otherwise, others feel that it is doubtful that a single cell extracted during the blastomere stage constitutes nor can create a life any more than during any stage following fertilization and replication from the initial single cell.[40]

## THE POLITICS OF STEM CELL RESEARCH

Just as the ethical and moral issues of stem cell research have not been resolved, the political debate over stem cell research rages as well. At the end of the 1992 presidential campaign, Bill Clinton announced his intention to overturn the de facto prohibition of research on human embryos that had been put in place by President George H.W. Bush. On June 10, 1993, the newly elected President Clinton signed legislation authorizing the NIH to begin to conduct and fund human embryo research. But, worrying that federal funds could be abused for research on human cloning, he issued an executive order in 1994, prohibiting the creation of human embryos for research purposes. To many ethicists, scientists, and politicians, this executive order was deemed insufficient to make sure that NIH considerable funds would not be misused. Therefore, in the summer of 1995, members of Congress decided to attach a rider to the Health and Human Services Appropriations Act that was used to fund the NIH each year. The "Dickey amendment," as it became known, prohibited the NIH from using appropriated funds for the creation of human embryos for research purposes. The amendment defined a human embryo as being an organism capable of becoming a human being when implanted in a uterus.[41] Using this very broad language, the act essentially prevented the use of federal funds for almost any research related to human embryonic stem cells.

In 1998, after the initial successes of the research groups from the University of Wisconsin and Johns Hopkins, the Clinton administration decided to re-evaluate its position on the support of embryonic stem cell research. The NIH requested a legal opinion from the Department of Health and Human Services (DHHS) on whether federal funds could be made available to researchers working with the human ES cells produced by the groups of Wisconsin and Johns Hopkins. In January of 1999, Harriet Rabb, the general counsel of DHHS, found that the Dickey amendment could not apply to human embryonic stem cells. The Dickey amendment officially defines a human embryo as being an *organism* capable of becoming a human being when implanted in a uterus. Becayse an ES cell cannot develop into a human being even when implanted in a uterus, Rabb determined that it could not be considered a human embryo. According to this logic, the DHHS maintained that despite the amendment, it could fund any research related to human ES cells, as long the cells were *initially* created with private funding.[42] That is, after careful consideration, DHHS concluded that because human pluripotent cells are not embryos, current federal law does not prohibit DHHS funds from being used for research utilizing these cells.

In April 1999, NIH director Harold Varmus appointed an oversight committee to begin drafting guidelines and provide oversight for the federal funding of ES cell research. The working group included scientists, clinicians, ethicists, lawyers, patients, and patient advocates. By February 2000, over 50,000 comments had been received by experts in fields as far ranging as medicine, philosophy, ethics, biology, and neuroscience. Finally, in the summer of 2000, NIH published the final set of guidelines, NIH Guidelines for Research Using Human Pluripotent Stem Cells, in the *Federal Register*, which became effective on August 25, 2000.[43] The purpose of the NIH Guidelines was to set forth procedures to help ensure that NIH-funded stem cell research was conducted in an ethical and legal manner. Among other stipulations, the NIH Guidelines prescribed that for studies using human pluripotent stem cells derived from human embryos, NIH funds may be used only if the cells were derived from frozen embryos that were created for the purpose of fertility treatment, were in excess of clinical need, and were obtained after the consent of the donating couple.

The Clinton administration's guidelines for stem cell research were actually relatively conservative in comparison to the policies of other developed countries. In accordance with the Dickey amendment, which had been renewed on every DHHS appropriations bill since 1997, the guidelines only allowed federal funding for studies using stem cells derived from embryos created for the purposes of in vitro fertilization, and only if they were in excess of the clinical need for such embryos. In addition, it was decided that the NIH could not fund any research that actually involved the derivation or creation of ES cells, because this was explicitly barred by the Dickey amendment.[44]

Furthermore, the Clinton administration decided to outlaw the use of NIH funds for research involving ES cells derived by using therapeutic cloning (somatic cell nuclear transfer, or SCNT), even if the actual derivation of the cells was performed with private funds.[45] SCNT is the only known technique that could potentially create embryonic stem cells that are genetically identical to an individual. That is, the cloned cell is used to create a stem cell line, not to create a new human being that would be a perfect genetic match for a patient. Stem cells that are created by this method would presumably avoid immune rejection, the primary concern of tissue transplantation. Without the ability to use therapeutic cloning, scientists utilizing federal funding would not be able to participate in research related to the "personalized medicine" that had become the ultimate goal for many stem cell researchers.

With the new guidelines in place, the NIH began to accept grant applications from research projects using human ES cells. The first review of these grants was supposed to occur by April 2001, several months after the Clinton administration left office. In mid-April, however, the DHHS decided to postpone the meeting until the incoming Bush administration could review the department's policies. After several months of review, on August 9, 2001, President George W. Bush announced the first federal funding of human embryonic stem cell research. Funding would however only be available to researchers using the seventy-eight human ES cell lines that had been created prior to that date. President Bush believed that the government could explore the promise and potential of stem cell research without crossing a fundamental moral line. Of the seventy-eight cell lines that were originally eligible for federal funding, only fifteen are currently available. The remainder of the eligible stem cell lines was either unavailable or unsuitable for research. With so few lines actually available, relatively few federal dollars have actually been spent on human stem cell research.

The President's Council on Bioethics issued a white paper on alternative sources of pluripotent stem cells in 2005.[46] Essentially, the council had no unanimous recommendations to make because so much needed to be done scientifically and because there are so many ethical considerations to be resolved. The council felt that is was a desirable goal to make an extra effort to seek out, assess, and find new ethical, uncontroversial methods of stem cell derivation. In essence, the council's report mirrors the ongoing debate in Congress and among private groups.

## WHO IS FUNDING STEM CELL RESEARCH?

Federal funding for biomedical research, done primarily through the NIH, is one of the most important sources of money for such research in the United States. Embryonic stem cell research, despite its potential, only gets 0.1% of federal biomedical research funding. And, of the $569 million spent on stem cell research in 2005, only $40 million was spent on *embryonic* stem cell research.[47] The vast majority of the money was used to support research on *adult* stem cells, which are currently believed to have far less long-term potential than embryonic stem cells. Moreover, the federal government will finance research only on stem cell lines created before August 9, 2001, from embryos left over from IVF treatment. The relative lack of federal funding for stem cell research has seriously undermined the ability of U.S. scientists to compete with researchers in countries more hospitable to this form of research. International scientists are currently racing ahead of U.S. scientists in research progress and scientific publishing primarily because of less restrictive policies regarding funding stem cell research.[48]

To be fair, the U.S. federal government has not outlawed any specific type of stem cell research per se as long as the research does not use federal funding. In fact, despite the rather stringent federal funding guidelines published in 2001, much work has been performed in the United States on stem cell research. Both state government and private funds have been used not only to create new stem cell lines from surplus embryos collected for IVF, embryos that otherwise would have been destroyed, but also to support research focusing on therapeutic cloning techniques. In fact, to make up for the strict federal regulations, some state governments have moved to increase their funding for embryonic stem cell research.

In 2004, the same year the Bush administration was elected to a second term in office, California passed proposition 71, an act that provided over $295 million a year for stem cell research projects.[49] Hoping that the proposition would make the state a hub of biomedical research, the plan was passed overwhelmingly by California voters. While it is an extremely bold initiative, this proposition does not support the use of state funds for any research involving the use of therapeutic cloning technologies. Following in California's footsteps, then-governor Richard J. Codey of New Jersey announced a statewide initiative to provide over $380 million to create a state-run foundation for stem cell research. Construction on the Stem Cell Institute of New Jersey was to have begun by the end of 2006.[50] Nevertheless, eleven state governments have banned all human embryo research, and two (Arkansas and Virginia) have prohibited both therapeutic and reproductive cloning. At present, in the remaining thirty-seven states, there are no laws specifically banning any form of stem cell research.

A showdown of sorts occurred in July 2006. Five years after President Bush initially opened the door to federal funding for stem cell research, albeit with strings attached, Congress was considering a bill that would loosen the carefully calibrated research restrictions outlined in 2001. Specifically, the bill would expand federal financing for embryonic stem cell research by allowing the government to pay for studies on stem cell lines that were derived from embryos stored at fertility clinics that were scheduled for destruction. The lack of consensus among the Republicans, in particular, on this issue provided the impetus for a loosening of current policy. Many in Congress, including the Majority Leader Bill Frist, publicly sided against the president by supporting embryonic stem cell research. Also, the American public supports federal funding of embryonic stem cell research by almost a two to one margin.[51] The bill passed and President Bush vetoed it.

A day after the President's veto, the Republican Governor of California, Arnold Schwarzenegger, authorized a $150 million loan from the state's general fund to pay for grants for stem cell research. In Illinois, the Democrat Governor, Rod Blagojevich, offered $5 million for similar grants. The issue of stem cell research has been infused into re-election campaigns across the country, and many Republicans are distancing themselves from the president on this issue.[52] More than one hundred bills have been considered by dozens of state legislatures, with one state (South Dakota) banning such research altogether. While California, Connecticut, Illinois, Maryland, and New Jersey have allocated state resources for this research, others have taken steps to support stem cell research without directly paying for the research.

While the debate rages, some scientists have expressed concern about individual states trying to mount efforts in absence of federal support. But, until the federal government's policy is changed, those in favor of stem cell research have to focus on state initiatives. As the Illinois governor said, "Investing in research that can save lives and prevent serious illnesses is more than a sound public health strategy, it's our moral obligation."[53]

## WHERE DO WE GO FROM HERE?

Few areas of biomedical science have aroused as much controversy as embryonic stem cell research. Since the derivation of the first human embryonic stem cells in 1998, the issue has been at the forefront of scientific, political, and ethical debate. Proponents tend to emphasize the considerable therapeutic potential of stem cell research, whereas opponents speak of the immorality of using human cells for this purpose. Yet, those individuals suffering from debilitating diseases for which stem cells may offer a cure, such as PD, diabetes, and spinal cord injuries, view the use of embryonic stem cells as the best means to treat or even cure their illness.

Stem cell research involves such unprecedented opportunities to improve medical science that it is hard not to be overwhelmed by its sheer potential. The major legal, ethical, religious, and political hurdles continue to fuel the debate. Both proponents and opponents make cogent arguments for and against embryonic stem cell research. What is needed is a scientific resolution to the moral dilemmas, with input from both science and medical ethics. Yet, given the scope of the issue, it is unlikely that the issue will be resolved quickly, and the broader application of embryonic stem cell research to those who could potentially benefit is still a hope and a dream.

# — 5 —

# Marijuana as Medicine:
# Science versus Politics

## WHAT'S IN A NAME?

The first known use of the name "marijuana" is attributed to Pancho Villa's supporters in Mexico in the late nineteenth century.[1] Today, there are countless names and terms for marijuana including pot, weed, grass, ganja, hash, and cannabis. In its more concentrated, resinous form, it is called hashish (hash, dope). Usually smoked as a cigarette (joint) or in a pipe (bong), it also can be smoked in a cigar that has been emptied of tobacco and refilled with marijuana (blunt). When smoked, marijuana has a distinctively pungent, sweet/sour odor. Marijuana also can be mixed in food and brewed as a tea.

Marijuana is a plant, more precisely a mix of flowers, stems, seeds, and leaves of the plant *Cannabis sativa*. Hemp is a common name for *Cannabis sativa* and is the name most used when this annual plant is grown for nondrug purposes; that is, fiber for rope, sacking, carpet, and textiles.[2] Hemp use dates back to the Stone Age as hemp fiber imprints have been found in pottery shards in China dating from over 10,000 years ago. But, hemp contains delta-9-tetrahydrocannabinol (THC), which is the psychoactive ingredient found in hashish and marijuana. THC stimulates a series of cellular reactions that lead to the high that users hope to experience when they smoke marijuana or hashish. The illegal widespread use of *Cannabis sativa* as a recreational drug overshadows the industrial (and legal) use of the plant.

Medical marijuana refers to the use of *Cannabis sativa* (THC in particular) as a therapeutic drug prescribed for a wide variety of therapeutic applications including relief from nausea and appetite loss, reduction of intraocular pressure, reduction of muscle spasms, and relief from chronic pain. While marijuana has been reported to offer relief of symptoms for AIDS patients, individuals undergoing chemotherapy, and those with multiple sclerosis (MS), it is not a completely benign substance. When smoked, marijuana can be as harmful as tobacco smoke. In addition, the plant contains a mixture of biologically active compounds that cannot be expected to provide a precisely defined drug effect.[3] For this reason, smoked marijuana for medical purposes may not be as safe as pharmaceutical medicines. Indeed, as will be discussed in this chapter, the evidence supporting the use of cannabis for medical purposes is mixed. Some claim that it is effective for a wide spectrum of medical problems, whereas others claim that it is not effective, and probably is harmful.

The history of the legitimate and legal medical uses of marijuana clearly shows how political ideology, rhetoric, and action impeded, in fact made almost impossible, scientific quantification of the risks and benefits of marijuana. How safe is medical marijuana? How valid are the arguments, pro and con, regarding the potential uses of marijuana? This chapter addresses the scientific and political issues of medical marijuana as debated in the United States over the decades.

## THE BIOLOGY OF MARIJUANA AND CANNABINOIDS

Marijuana is a complex mixture of over 400 biochemically active compounds of which THC is the primary active component responsible for the plant's mind-altering effect. Researchers in Israel, in 1964, were the first to identify THC as the main psychoactive cannabinoid in marijuana.[4] The concentration of THC and the other cannabinoids in marijuana varies greatly depending on the growing conditions and processing after harvesting. Usually, the concentration of THC ranges from 0.3% to 4% by weight, but specially grown and selected marijuana can contain 15% or more of THC.[5]

There are approximately sixty other chemicals in marijuana called cannabinoids (compounds that have some of the properties of THC but cause less psychoactive effects), which appear in no other plant. The inherently variable potency of the plant material complicates describing the clinical pharmacology of marijuana, and that marijuana is smoked or eaten in more or less its natural form also complicates matters. Logically, the route of administration (smoked or eaten, for example) will affect absorption and metabolism. When marijuana is smoked, THC rapidly passes from the lungs into the bloodstream and then throughout the body. Oral ingestion is quite different as maximum THC blood levels are reached one to three hours after eating, and the onset of psychoactive and other pharmacological effects are slower than the effect one gets after smoking marijuana. Despite the potent psychoactivity and pharmacological actions of THC on the body, cannabinoids have remarkably low lethal toxicity.

While it is not well understood how THC acts on brain cells or what general areas of the brain are most affected by THC, it appears that THC connects to specific sites (cannabinoid receptors) on nerve cells in the brain. Many cannabinoid receptors have been identified in the parts of the brain that influence pleasure, memory, thought, concentration, sensory and time perception, and coordinated movement.[6] Different cannabinoids appear to have different effects on the body, and there are a variety of mechanisms through which they can influence human physiology. The differing mechanisms through which cannabinoids influence human physiology underlies the variety of potential therapeutic uses for drugs that might act selectively on different cannabinoid systems.[7] However, more research is needed to understand the physiological effects of synthetic and plant-derived cannabinoids, as well as the effects attributed to THC.

## A BIT OF HISTORY

Cannabis has been used for medicinal purposes for tens of thousands of years. Its therapeutic use was first recorded in 2737 BC in China under the emperor Shen Nung. The medical use of cannabis was also known India, Greece, Egypt, and Persia.[8] Apparently ancient doctors used it to treat a variety of illnesses and ailments and prescribed it as a pain reliever.[9] There is evidence that during the Bronze Age (circa 1400 BC), there was a thriving drug trade in hashish and opium throughout the eastern Mediterranean. Indeed, throughout the centuries travelers and traders carried the knowledge of cannabis to far-off places.

In the early seventeenth century in America, the first marijuana law was enacted at Jamestown Colony mandating ("ordering") farmers to grow hemp.[10] Massachusetts, Connecticut, and the Chesapeake Colonies also passed "must grow" laws. The Pilgrims planted cannabis throughout New England to be used primarily for fibers.

During the nineteenth century, cannabis was used as a medicine in most parts of the world; specifically, it was used as the primary painkiller until the invention of aspirin. British doctors recommended it as an appetite stimulant, analgesic, muscle relaxant, anticonvulsant, and hypnotic. Marijuana and hashish extracts were the most prescribed medicines in the United States at this time,[11] and in 1870, cannabis was listed as a medicine in the *U.S. Pharmacopoeia*. But, by the end of the nineteenth century, the medical use of cannabis declined as the medical profession began to prescribe other medications that were considered to be superior. Apparently cannabis as a medicine was disputed, and its image as an intoxicant didn't help matters.

In the early twentieth century, the U.S. Congress passed a series of laws and acts that focused primarily on restricting the sale and use of narcotics and eventually on defining the legality of marijuana. One of the first, the Pure Food and Drug Act of 1906, banned the interstate transportation of adulterated or mislabeled food and drugs and set standards of quality and truth in labeling. Importantly, the patent medicine industry now was required to list the ingredients in their products, which rapidly led to the demise of this industry. The

U.S. Congress passed the Harrison Act of 1914, one of the most influential legislative acts concerning drug importation, distribution, and use, which became the standard for the basis of narcotic regulation in the United States for the next fifty years. The act gave the federal government the authority to raise revenue and to tax and regulate the distribution and sale of narcotics. While perhaps initially intended to establish an orderly marketing of opium, morphine, and heroin, the law ended up prohibiting the supplying of narcotics to addicts, even to those who had a doctor's prescription. In addition, the law permitted the arrest and imprisonment of physicians who wrote such prescriptions. The act ultimately served to make the nonmedical use of morphine and cocaine illegal.

Despite Congressional action, by 1920 in the United States an illicit drug economy was thriving (primarily on the sale of cocaine and heroin). Taking action again, Congress passed the Jones–Miller Act of 1922, which imposed fines of up to $5,000 and prison sentences for up to ten years for anyone found guilty of importing narcotics. All this act seemed to do was increase the price of heroin and cocaine, and it had little influence on the illicit drug trade. Also in 1922, the Narcotic Drug Import and Export Act was passed by the U.S. Congress and was intended to eliminate the use of narcotics except for legitimate use.

In addition to Congressional actions to stem the use and sale of narcotics, the states were actively involved in regulation. Utah, in 1915, was the first to pass an anti-marijuana law. California, Texas, Louisiana, Nevada, Oregon, Washington, and New York followed suit to outlaw cannabis. Other countries, too, were taking action: in Canada, cannabis was added to the schedule of prohibited drugs of the Opium and Narcotic Drug Act and cannabis was declared a narcotic in 1924. In the United Kingdom, cannabis was made illegal under the Dangerous Drugs Act of 1928.

By the mid-1930s, cannabis, now described as a "narcotic poison," was used very little in medical practice. It was considered unstable and unreliable, and the consensus was that there were other drugs that could be used to relieve pain better and safer. Focusing specifically on marijuana, Congress passed the Marijuana Tax Act of 1937, which did not ban marijuana outright, but made it difficult for physicians to prescribe it for medical purposes. The act made it illegal to import marijuana into the United States, and also imposed an occupational excise tax on dealers and a transfer tax on dealings in marijuana. Marijuana was placed in the same category as cocaine and opium products. Despite the legal restrictions, marijuana use was not curbed.

One of the most vociferous opponents of marijuana was Harry J. Anslinger, the head of the Federal Bureau of Narcotics and Dangerous Drugs. During the 1940s, while some research was focused on assessing marijuana's therapeutic applications, Anslinger threatened to send the researchers to jail if his personal permission was not first obtained. He used his full power to halt virtually all research into marijuana and blackmailed the American Medical Association into denouncing the New York Academy of Medicine and its doctors for the research they had performed.[12] Still on his crusade in the early 1960s, Anslinger was instrumental in getting the United Nations Treaty 406 Single Convention on Narcotic Drugs of 1961 passed. This treaty sought to coordinate international narcotic control and to outlaw cannabis use and cannabis cultivation worldwide.[13] It essentially made cannabis equal to opium and cocaine. Ironically, President John F. Kennedy, who used cannabis for pain relief, fired Anslinger, but the damage was done. Marijuana, opium, and cocaine were viewed as being equally dangerous.

Despite the political machinations going on in the first half of the twentieth century, and despite the fact that marijuana was officially removed from the *U.S. Pharmacopoeia* in 1941, research was being conducted in several countries to assess marijuana's medicinal effects. For example, The Wooton Report (United Kingdom), issued in 1968, concluded that the long-term consumption of cannabis in moderate doses had no harmful effects.[14] Nevertheless, the U.S. Congress, clearly not impressed by the British report's conclusion, passed the Comprehensive Drug Abuse Prevention and Control Act of 1970 (U.S. Controlled Substances Act), which served to repeal the Marijuana Tax Act of 1937 and consolidate over fifty federal narcotic, marijuana, and dangerous drug laws into one law that was designed to control the legitimate drug industry and to curtail importation and distribution of illicit drugs in the United States.[15] Marijuana continued to be grouped with heroin, cocaine, and other illicit narcotics.

A defined a schedule of controlled substances (Schedule I–V) was created. All substances listed are available by prescription except for Schedule I drugs (substances that have no accepted medical utility but have substantial potential for abuse), which could not be prescribed unless the physician and the patient were participants in an approved research project. Marijuana was listed as a Schedule I drug, along with heroin and other hallucinogens. As a point of reference, Schedule II drugs (substances having a high abuse liability but also having some accepted medical purpose) included morphine and cocaine. What this meant was that physicians were permitted to prescribe cocaine and morphine, but not marijuana.

Also in the early 1970s, Congress passed the Drug Abuse Office and Treatment Act of 1972, which created the Special Action Office for Drug Abuse Prevention within the Executive Office of the President. It was the Carter administration's position to allow states to decriminalize possession of small amounts of marijuana for personal use. There was an effort to distinguish between narcotics and marijuana, and decriminalization was a state-by-state choice that was not to be mandated by the federal government. But, there apparently was a huge difference in opinion as to how to regulate marijuana. Eleven states decriminalized possession of small amounts of marijuana for personal use during the 1970s, and New Mexico, Illinois, Texas, Georgia, Minnesota, Rhode Island, South Carolina, New York, and New Jersey enacted laws that authorized a medical marijuana research program for patients with cancer and, in some states, for patients with glaucoma.[16] While the respective state legislatures took such action, no program was ever operational!

Meanwhile, early research on the medicinal properties of marijuana showed that for many patients, cannabis was associated with a reduction in pain; a decrease in intraocular pressure (high intraocular pressure can cause blindness in glaucoma patients); had an effect on alleviating and mitigating muscle spasms, tics, and spasticity; and had antiemetic (anti-nausea) properties. The *New York Times* even reported in a 1976 article that scientists could find nothing really harmful about marijuana.[17] Perhaps ironically, the substantial increase in the number of recreational marijuana users in the 1970s contributed to the rediscovery of marijuana's medical uses. As word spread, many more individuals started self-medicating with marijuana. Yet, despite the anecdotal stories of marijuana's therapeutic value, and despite some studies showing the potential value of marijuana as a medicine, the federal government continued its opposition to the medicinal uses of marijuana.

One of the early court cases focusing on the medical use of marijuana was heard in 1976. Robert Randall, who suffered from glaucoma, was arrested for cultivating his own marijuana. He employed a little-used Common Law Doctrine of Necessity to defend himself against criminal charges of marijuana cultivation. In *United States v. Randall*, it was ruled that Randall's use of marijuana constituted a "medical necessity," and as a result of this ruling a procedure was devised to allow patients to receive medical marijuana from the U.S. government.[18] The court ruling forced the government to find a way to provide Mr. Randall and others with marijuana, leading to the establishment of the Investigational New Drug (IND) compassionate access program. Marijuana was grown on a government farm in Mississippi and could only be obtained from the National Institute on Drug Abuse (NIDA). Since its inception in 1974, NIDA has been the only legal source for cannabis in the United States.[19]

While the 1970s could be characterized as being more open-minded about the medical properties of marijuana, the 1980s saw a continuation of the federal government's efforts to restrict and penalize medical marijuana use. The Reagan administration's position on medical marijuana differed significantly from that of the Carter administration. For example, the Reagan administration went so far as to call on all American universities and researchers to destroy all 1966–76 cannabis research. This censorship was strongly rebuffed and the administration backed down; however, marijuana remained listed as a Schedule I narcotic. The 1980s saw the passage of four major anti-drug bills:

- The Comprehensive Crime Control Act of 1984 (broadened criminal and civil asset forfeiture laws and increased federal criminal sanctions for drug offenses)
- The 1986 Anti-Drug Abuse Act (provided more money for prevention and treatment but restored mandatory prison sentences for large-scale distribution of marijuana)

- The 1988 Anti-Drug Abuse Amendment Act (increased the sanctions for crimes related to drug trafficking and raised federal penalties for marijuana possession, cultivation, and trafficking)
- The Crime Control Act of 1990 (focused on supply reduction and law enforcement)

At the same time that Congress was passing restrictive laws, the Drug Enforcement Administration's Chief Administrative Law Judge ruled in 1988 that marijuana in its natural form was one of the safest therapeutically active substances, and it would be unreasonable, arbitrary, and capricious for the Drug Enforcement Administration (DEA) to continue to prohibit marijuana use when prescribed by a physician for those who would benefit from this substance.[20]

Under the Clinton administration, a petition for the rescheduling of cannabis was made to the U.S. District Court in the mid-1990s. The request was to have marijuana and all cannabinoids removed from Schedule I and II because it was argued that they do not have the abuse potential as required for inclusion in those schedules. The Court rejected this petition but did produce a five-part revised formulation for determining whether a drug has an accepted medical use: (1) the drug's chemistry must be known and reproducible, (2) there have to have been adequate safety studies, (3) there have to have been conducted well-controlled studies proving efficacy, (4) the drug must be accepted by qualified experts, and (5) scientific evidence must be widely available. In 2001, another petition to reschedule marijuana to permit medical use was also denied.

While the federal policy towards marijuana clearly made little distinction between narcotics, cocaine, and marijuana, individual states continued to take a more liberal view of marijuana. Voters in Arizona in 1996 approved Proposition 200, an initiative endorsing the legal use of marijuana under a doctor's supervision, and voters in California approved a similar initiative (Proposition 215). A special hearing of the Senate Judiciary Committee was called at the request of Senator Orrin Hatch of Utah to denounce the passage of these initiatives. The federal government's position was clear: the federal government could take both administrative and criminal actions against doctors who violated the terms of their DEA's drug registrations to prescribe controlled substances. The federal government's stance was that the propositions didn't change anything.[21]

Despite the admission by President Clinton that in his youth he smoked marijuana, but did not inhale, his administration went so far as to propose instituting criminal prosecution of physicians who prescribed marijuana in California and Arizona and excluding these physicians from the Medicare and Medicaid programs. In response, opponents of the Clinton administration proposal called for a comprehensive review of marijuana's medical benefits and risks by the National Academy of Science's Institute of Medicine (IOM).

The IOM report, published in 1999, was the most comprehensive summary and analysis of the topic at the time. The IOM panel recommended that there were some limited circumstances in which smoking marijuana for medical use would be beneficial. Specifically, the accumulated evidence indicated a potential therapeutic value particularly for pain relief, control of nausea and vomiting, and for appetite stimulation. The data further supported the conclusion that the adverse effects of marijuana were within the range of effects tolerated for other medications. The report also addressed the question of whether the medical uses of marijuana would lead to an increase in use among the general population. The conclusion was that there were no data to support such concerns.[22]

While state action and public opinion clearly were in opposition to the federal government's anti-marijuana crusade, members of Congress continued to introduce legislation to sanction physicians who prescribed or recommended medical marijuana use. The then-editor of the respected *New England Journal of Medicine*, Dr. Jerome Kassirer, wrote that the federal policy prohibiting physicians from prescribing marijuana to seriously ill patients is misguided, heavy-handed, and inhumane.[23] More lawsuits by groups of physicians, health organizations, and patients were filed challenging the federal government's refusal to allow physicians to prescribe medical marijuana in states that permitted them to do so. The continued disconnect between the federal policy and state policy could not be clearer.

Protests against the federal policy continued into the twenty-first century. In 2002, federal agents frequently raided medical marijuana suppliers and clinics in California. Two medical marijuana users filed suit against federal authorities in an effort to try to stop government raids. Plaintiffs Angel McClary Raich and Diane Monson, who said that they required medical marijuana to help ease the pain of their illnesses, filed suit to prevent federal officials from arresting them for using marijuana under the state's 1996 law allowing medical use. Both had followed their doctors' advice to use marijuana to alleviate symptoms of their medical condition (Ms. Raich had an inoperable brain tumor and other health problems and Ms. Monson had a painful degenerative spine disease). A 2003 federal appeals court ruling in the patients' favor was quickly appealed to the Supreme Court, which heard oral arguments in the case (*Ashcroft v. Raich*) in November 2004.

In June 2005, relying on the "commerce clause" in the constitution that gives Congress the power to regulate interstate commerce, the Supreme Court ruled six to three that the federal Controlled Substances Act trumps state laws when it comes to the regulation of controlled substances. Federal authorities may prosecute sick people who smoke marijuana on doctor's orders, and state medical marijuana laws don't protect users from a federal ban on the drug. The decision was a stinging defeat for marijuana advocates and those eleven states that had passed laws to allow doctors to prescribe marijuana for medical purposes.[24] The court ruling continued to put the federal government at odds with many in the scientific community and with public opinion.

*Ashcroft v. Raich* was one of the most closely watched Supreme Court suits. A ruling against the federal government would have had far-reaching legal implications but also would have been a major blow to aggressive George W. Bush White House anti-marijuana policies. What the case didn't do was settle the question of whether marijuana is an effective medicine at all, or if so, whether voters or even state legislatures should be allowed to take on medical treatment questions usually reserved for the FDA.

In summary, over the past decades, legal and legislative actions highlight the twisted path of the legal use of marijuana for medical purposes. Legislation made very little distinction between narcotics, cocaine, and marijuana; federal law did not recognize any distinction between marijuana and other illicit substances. While the 1937 Marijuana Tax Act effectively stopped physicians from using marijuana as medicine, the 1970 Controlled Substances Act placed marijuana as a Schedule I drug, and subsequent efforts to move marijuana from Schedule I to another schedule repeatedly failed. Often, state regulations differed sharply with congressional action as numerous states allowed for the medical use of marijuana.

The U.S. federal government does not, and never has, recognized legitimate medical uses of marijuana. Throughout time, however, cannabis use, as a recreational drug or as a medical product, persisted. Most of the legislative and judicial actions in the twentieth and twenty-first centuries in the United States clearly had a political bias and were not based on empirical evidence. What do the studies show about the efficacy and safety of marijuana? To what extent is marijuana a valid therapeutic agent? Is the legal ban on medical marijuana warranted? To what extent did politics dictate policy? Was the federal government correct in taking such a strong stand against the use of marijuana for medical purposes?

The following provides a succinct summary of published research. The emphasis is on evidence-based medicine as opposed to opinion-based medicine.

## MARIJUANA'S THERAPEUTIC EFFECTS

The therapeutic potential of medical marijuana and cannabinoids, the active ingredient in cannabis, have many distinct pharmacological properties including analgesic, anti-nausea, and neuroprotective.[25] Research since the mid-1990s as summarized in the Institute of Medicine's comprehensive report, *Marijuana and Medicine: Assessing the Science Base*[26] has helped clarify a number of issues concerning medical marijuana's benefits and risks. There was accumulating evidence to suggest that medical marijuana could be beneficial for those suffering from a variety of diseases such as MS and HIV, as well as for those undergoing chemotherapy. However, it must be stated that many of the studies are methodologically weak: small study sample, not randomized placebo-controlled clinical trials comparing conventional treatments to medical marijuana, doses not standardized among studies, and so on. Further complicating the issue is the fact that actual absorbed doses of THC from smoked marijuana vary greatly among individuals. Smoking behavior is not easily quantified and puff and inhalation volume differs from person to person. Indeed, a smoker's experience is probably an important determinant of dose actually absorbed.[27] Oral use of marijuana, too, is also variable because of the metabolism of the drug.

## SIDE EFFECTS AND RISKS ASSOCIATED WITH MARIJUANA

Although scientific studies (mainly based on smoked marijuana) indicate the potential therapeutic value of cannabinoid drugs, primarily THC, for pain relief, control of nausea and vomiting, and appetite stimulation, marijuana is not a benign substance. The primary acute adverse effect of marijuana is diminished psychomotor performance (don't operate heavy machinery or make important decisions!). For many, there are psychological effects such as anxiety reduction and euphoria, which some could argue can be therapeutically helpful. Short-term effects of marijuana can include problems with memory, distorted perception, difficulty in thinking and problem solving, loss of coordination, and increased heart rate.

Although few users develop a dependence on marijuana, there are known adverse risks: marijuana smoking is associated with abnormalities of cells lining the human respiratory tract that can lead to an increased risk of lung damage, respiratory disease, and cancer. Frequent marijuana smokers may develop many of the same respiratory problems as tobacco smokers (cough, phlegm production, obstructed airways).[28–31] Marijuana has the potential to increase blood pressure, heart rate, and decrease the oxygen-carrying capacity of blood, which could increase the risk of heart attack in some individuals.[32] In addition, a distinctive marijuana withdrawal syndrome, characterized by restlessness, irritability, insomnia, sleep disturbance, nausea, and cramping, has been noted in some users, but it is generally mild and short lived. A potentially serious side effect of marijuana use is related to its immunosuppressive effect. Clearly, this effect would be more serious for cancer patients who already have immune suppression as a result of their chemotherapy treatment.

Depression, anxiety, paranoia, and personality disturbances have been associated with frequent marijuana use.[33–35] Heavy marijuana users have more trouble sustaining and shifting their attention and in registering, organizing, and using information compared with infrequent users and nonusers.[36] Especially among older individuals, the psychoactive effects of cannabis (mind-altering side effects including euphoria, relaxation, and drowsiness) are not always appreciated or tolerated well.

Heavy marijuana use can lead to problems including an adverse impact on memory and learning, trouble sustaining attention, and trouble learning. But, long-term marijuana use is not addicting, although there have been anecdotal reports that some long-term marijuana users may exhibit craving and withdrawal symptoms that make it hard to stop using the drug.[37] At this time, there are no medications available to treat marijuana abuse although as more is understood about the workings of THC receptors, there is the possibility of developing a medication that would block the intoxicating effects of THC by lessening or eliminating the appeal of the drug.

Of course not every user will experience adverse side effects from smoking or ingesting marijuana. Certainly a person's age, immune status, disease status, frequency of use, how marijuana is used, and the like must be taken into account.

That being said, how valid are the therapeutic claims of medical marijuana?

## Pain Control

Chronic pain has been described as one of the most common reasons for therapeutic use of marijuana, but the "evidence" that medical marijuana or cannabinoids have analgesic efficacy is based largely on low-quality studies such as anecdotal reports, self reported surveys, and case series. From a scientific perspective, results of such studies are not very generalizable or representative and must be viewed with caution. The best way to establish whether cannabis is an effective and safe treatment option for pain management is to conduct a randomized double blind clinical trial.

Campbell and colleagues[38] conducted a systematic review of randomized, clinical trials published between 1975 and 1997 whose outcomes were pain intensity scores, pain relief scores, and adverse effects. Twenty randomized, controlled trials were identified of which eleven were excluded because of methodological problems. Of the remaining nine trials (222 patients), five related to cancer pain, two to chronic nonmalignant pain, and two to acute postoperative pain. No randomized, controlled trial evaluated the effects of marijuana or other inhaled or smoked cannabinoids per se, rather four different cannabinoids were tested, including an oral THC 5–20 mg, and were compared with oral codeine 50–120 mg and oral secobarbital 50 mg. Findings from this systematic review showed that cannabinoids are no more effective than codeine in controlling pain and often had depressant effects on the central nervous system, thus limiting their use for some individuals. The researchers found insufficient evidence to support the use of cannabinoids for pain relief or pain management given that there are effective treatments for pain available.

Cannabis has been reported (anecdotally) as being beneficial for pain relief (diffuse nerve pain–polyneuropathy) among some HIV patients.[39] While there are few methodologically sound studies looking at marijuana as an analgesic among HIV patients, one study of 565 patients found that of the 27% who used marijuana to treat their symptoms, pain relief was significant.[40] Another small-scale study of sixteen HIV-infected patients with neuropathy found that smoking three marijuana cigarettes each day for seven days showed a 30% reduction in average daily pain.[41] But, much more research would be needed before one could state that cannabis is an effective agent to control pain among HIV patients. That is, randomized, clinical trials comparing conventional pain treatments with cannabis for relief of pain associated with HIV are needed.

Other studies have looked at marijuana's potential to alleviate pain associated with MS. A double-blind, placebo-controlled trial looking specifically at reduction of pain among twenty-four patients with MS compared placebo with dronabinol 10 mg daily (Marinol, an oral synthetic THC approved by the FDA in 1985. Solvay Pharmaceuticals Inc., Marietta, GA). Findings showed that dronabinol had a modest but clinically relevant analgesic effect on central pain, but this was a very small study and results must be interpreted with caution. There were adverse events noted more frequently with dronabinol than with placebo.[42] Clearly, more research needed to be done to assess marijuana and dronabinol's benefits for patients with MS.

## Control of Nausea and Vomiting

There has been a lot of research conducted on the use of cannabinoids for chemotherapy-related nausea and vomiting. The potential seriousness of the problem of chemotherapy-induced nausea, and the fact that some cancer patients do not benefit from antiemetic pharmaceuticals, provided the impetus for oncologists to focus on the antiemetic properties of cannabinoids. The results from numerous clinical trials showed that THC is at least equivalent in effectiveness to antiemetic drugs. Given the wide variety of patients included in these trials, including different age groups, different cancers, different chemotherapeutic agents, and the variety of different antiemetics with which THC has been compared, the research findings showing the benefit of THC as an antiemetic are even more impressive.

## Glaucoma

Glaucoma is the third-leading cause of blindness in the United States and is characterized by increased pressure in the eyeball, which can lead to loss of vision. In the early 1970s, research showed that smoking marijuana reduced pressure in the eyes (lowered intraocular pressure) in people with normal pressure and those with glaucoma, although exactly how marijuana produced this effect is not clear.[43] The duration of action of marijuana after smoking was relative short (3–4 hours). More recent research has shown that smoking marijuana resulted in an average of a 25% reduction of intraocular pressure; however, not every participant experienced this reduction. Only 60%–65% had this effect.[44] There also were side effects caused by marijuana, including reduction in tears and orthostatic hypotension.

Presently, the consensus is that marijuana does not offer any advantages over currently available glaucoma treatments, and whether it is useful when used in combination with standard therapies has yet to be determined.[45] There are many available agents for treatment, and these topical preparations seem to control intraocular pressure well.

## MS

Research has focused on the effectiveness of cannabinoids in the treatment of tremors, spasticity, and muscle spasms associated with MS and other neurodegenerative diseases.[46,47] MS is an immune-mediated disease of the central nervous system. Some sufferers become massively disabled, while others can live their entire lives with minimal or no disability. A large placebo-controlled, double-blinded clinical trial conducted in Britain looked at the effect of marijuana extracts on MS symptoms and found that marijuana resulted in subjective improvements in spasticity, spasms, sleep, and pain.[48] However, there were more episodes of dizziness/light-headedness, dry mouth, and gastrointestinal symptoms in the treatment group.

A systematic review of fifteen clinical trials was assessed, and of this, two large trials found that cannabinoids were significantly better than placebo in managing spasticity in MS patients.[49] But, trials are particularly difficult to design, and those that have been conducted involved small number of patients and the assessment of spasticity and pain tended to be subjective. The better-designed studies have not demonstrated objective improvement in MS symptoms.[50] A large, randomized trial comparing oral THC, oral cannabis extract, and placebo showed no effect on spasticity based on an objective scale despite participants reporting fewer spasms and less pain.[51]

## HIV/AIDS

Although antiretroviral therapy has helped increased survival significantly, there also is a need to manage symptoms and side effects of this long-term drug therapy. Cannabis has been reported anecdotally as being beneficial for a number of common complications of HIV including poor appetite and pain caused by HIV-related peripheral neuropathy. One British study designed to measure the patterns and prevalence of marijuana use in patients presenting at a large HIV clinic found that 27% of the 523 respondents reported using marijuana for treating symptoms. While the majority of users reported reduction in muscle and nerve pain, nausea, depression, and an improvement in appetite, almost half reported associated memory deterioration.[52]

It has been known that there is a strong relationship between marijuana and dronabinol and increased appetite leading to weight gain.[53] A study conducted at San Francisco General Hospital found that patients using marijuana gained more weight than those receiving a placebo.[54] Other small-scale studies done in the 1980s and 1990s also showed similar results.

In summary, while there are numerous anecdotal reports of the "benefits" of marijuana (oral or smoked), there is a paucity of clinical trials and studies that would provide more definitive findings about the benefits and the risks of marijuana. Many of the studies cited herein report that many users reported that their symptoms improved after using marijuana, but some also reported adverse side effects such as memory deterioration, dizziness, and loss of coordination. Smoking marijuana carries its own set of risks. The purported benefits of marijuana have to be compared with the risks. Longer-term studies with larger study populations need to be conducted in to better determine the effectiveness of marijuana for medical purposes.

## PUBLIC OPINION VERSUS GOVERNMENT ACTION

Before the 2005 Supreme Court ruling, there was wide support for ending the prohibition of medical marijuana both among the medical community and the public. A CNN/Time poll conducted in 2002 found that 80% of Americans believed that adults should be allowed to legally use marijuana for medical purposes if their doctor prescribes it, and a 2004 poll taken by the American Association of Retired Persons showed that 72% of its members thought that people could use marijuana for medical purposes if their doctor recommended it.[55,56] Numerous professional organizations have publicly supported the legal use of marijuana for medical purposes.[57] As discussed earlier, state governments, too, have been more liberal than the federal government allowing marijuana to be prescribed by physicians for medical use. Indeed, state governments have been stymied by the federal government's legislative acts prohibiting the use of marijuana for medical purposes. The National Institute on Drug Abuse, the only legal source of marijuana for clinical research in the United States, consistently made it difficult (perhaps impossible) for researchers to obtain marijuana for clinical studies.

Efforts to bring change through the court system were not very successful because the courts tended to defer to the Drug Enforcement Agency whose actions have kept marijuana illegal in the United States. And now, the 2005 Supreme Court ruling probably makes the issue moot at this point in time.

While marijuana possession and supply are illegal in the United States, the United Kingdom, and Canada, the politico–legal stance in the United States differs from that in the other two countries. As of this writing, the British government has reclassified cannabis as a low-risk class C drug, and Canada allows legal procurement for individuals with demonstrable medical need. The Canadian government in 2001 passed the Marijuana Medical Access Regulation, which clearly outlines the circumstances and manner in which marijuana can be used therapeutically. Both Canada and the United Kingdom also sponsor research on marijuana's therapeutic benefits and risks. In contrast, the U.S. government has consistently refused to change its policy and repeatedly insisted that the evidence of marijuana's safety and efficacy is inadequate.

Based on what is known about marijuana's potential as a therapeutic agent, one could question why the U.S. federal government and the U.S. Supreme Court took such a hard stance against the use of marijuana for medical purposes. Whereas the option of prescribing and using marijuana for medical purposes has been blocked by court decree, physicians can prescribe morphine and other narcotics. Unlike many other psychoactive drugs, marijuana now cannot be prescribed to patients even in cases where physicians believe that it would be beneficial. The reasons for this prohibition are clearly politically ideological, but what was the basis for this ideology? Was there fear that individuals would abuse marijuana for nonmedical purposes if it were legally available?

Was refusing to remove marijuana as a Schedule I drug really warranted based on the evidence? Did the federal government go too far by having physicians who prescribed marijuana and patients who used it as a therapeutic treatment arrested and prosecuted? Does the evidence about marijuana's benefits and risks really warrant such action? Marijuana is not habit forming, unlike heroin or cocaine. Nobody has died from an overdose of marijuana. Marijuana produces no unacceptable long-term risks to its users. The evidence is clear on this.

Public opinion has consistently supported the legalization of marijuana for medical purposes, and marijuana has been shown (to some degree) to have medical value. Unfortunately, clinical research on the potential therapeutic uses for marijuana has been difficult, if not impossible to undertake, because of the federal government's actions despite the call for such research by scientists. Seriously ill people who had benefited from using marijuana must now find other means of controlling their pain, nausea, or muscle spasms. Although the scientific evidence of marijuana's therapeutic benefits is equivocal, for some diseases and conditions relief of symptoms from marijuana use was evident.

To answer unresolved issues regarding marijuana's effectiveness as a therapeutic, future studies will have to be conducted in countries where the politico–legal climate is more hospitable. But, it will be very important for these studies to be designed well and the outcomes carefully evaluated in a rigorous way. Other countries will have to lead the way as it is now impossible for such studies to be conducted in the United States. Perhaps in the case of medical marijuana, the U.S. federal government and the American courts overstepped their bounds, relying more on political expediencies than on research findings.

# — 6 —

# The Quintessential Catch-22:
# The U.S. Approach to Needle Exchange
# in HIV AIDS Prevention

## with Ivan Ip, MPH

The history of needle exchange programs (NEPs), particularly in the United States, is a clear example of how politics can run roughshod over science. Even though the scientific research uniformly showed that providing clean needles to injection drug users is an effective means of reducing the spread of human immunodeficiency virus (HIV) and hepatitis C virus, barriers to developing such exchange programs effectively prevented this public health measure from being implemented on a wide scale. In this chapter, we discuss the story behind the federal ban for funding NEPs and the implications of this policy.

### WHAT ARE NEEDLE EXCHANGE PROGRAMS INTENDED TO DO?

NEPs, or syringe exchange programs (SEPs), provide sterile syringes in exchange for used syringes to reduce transmission of HIV and other bloodborne infections associated with reuse of contaminated syringes by injection/intravenous drug users (IDUs). Often these programs provide other public health services, such as HIV testing and risk-reduction education, and make referrals to drug treatment and detoxification programs, social services agencies, and primary health care centers. Minorities are most severely affected by the lack of access to sterile syringes; the data are very clear that AIDS and HIV infection are disproportionately higher among African Americans and Hispanics compared with Whites. Injection drug use is a leading cause of infection in both men and women of color. Clearly, a program to help stop the transmission of bloodborne infection would be extremely beneficial both on an individual and societal level.

Today in the United States, 185 NEPs exist in more than 102 cities in 36 states, distributing more than 24.9 million syringes annually.[1] While many states and municipalities have taken action to improve access to sterile syringes, the actual possession, distribution, and sale of syringes is a criminal offense. Basically, the legality of the programs often depends on a country-by-county certification of a State of Emergency that must be regularly renewed. While some law enforcement agencies recognize the benefits of NEPs, there are numerous cases of police harassment of NEP workers and clients. Zero-tolerance drug policies, which in many states criminalize both the possession of syringes and the distribution of sterile syringes, exacerbate the problem.

The political inaction against national liberalization of needle access policies, in spite of widespread scientific support, brings to light values, beliefs, and attitudes that have left thousands of drug addicts dead and thousands of others at unnecessarily high risk of acquiring an incurable disease. Despite the knowledge that HIV transmission is best prevented by avoiding contaminated needle use, IDUs in most areas of the United States continue to lack access to clean needles. Even with the support of various prominent organizations, such as the American Public Health Association, the World Health Organization, and the Centers for Disease Control and Prevention (CDC), NEPs remain restricted by broader political forces that often have overtly undermined the mission of saving lives. A federal ban on government funding for NEPs prevails after seventeen years of continued protests by numerous advocacy leaders.[2] Indeed, the legal status of 21% of existing NEP operations remains questionable, and there has been evidence of police harassment at some NEPs, including those that have been tolerated by the local officials.[3] In addition, there have been reports of individuals risking arrest on the way to and from a needle exchange site.

## A DISEASE OF TRAGEDY

As with many things in life, timing is everything. In the United States, the beginning of the AIDS epidemic unfortunately emerged just months after Ronald Reagan was inaugurated. Not long after taking office, Reagan pronounced that, "It is my intention to curb the size and influence of the federal establishment and to demand recognition of the distinction between the powers granted to the federal government and those reserved to the states or to the people."[4] Determined to trim the nation's budget deficit, the actor-turned-governor of the state of California and now President of the United States was intent on reducing funding for virtually every branch of government. Within months, many Health and Human Services programs, such as the Indian Health Service and the Office of Refugee Health, were eliminated. Budgets for Medicaid and Medicare, the safety net healthcare system for the indigent and elderly, were slashed from $1.9 billion in 1981 to $1.4 billion in 1982.

Politically, the promise of fiscal responsibility won the support of many voters. However, the cutback left most of the U.S. public health system weakened and underfunded. As doctors in New York, Los Angeles, San Francisco, and Washington, DC, raised alarm over the increasing number of deaths among patients suffering from severe immune suppression, the public health care system, reeling from the cuts, was hampered in its effort to do much about the situation. Despite exhortations of the nation's leading health experts, funding for the scientific research that could afford some insight into the intricacies of this growing puzzling disease remained scarce. Support to agencies responsible for the surveillance and public education necessary for any kind of effective preventive intervention was vastly inadequate. So little attention was given to AIDS by the Reagan administration that five years into the crisis, in 1986, the Institute of Medicine called the government's effort to stimulate scientific AIDS research "woefully inadequate."[5] Complicating matters was the widespread ignorance, fear, and bigotry against those sick and dying of AIDS.

Among the early AIDS victims were homosexual men and drug addicts, two groups disliked by politicians, many of whom viewed AIDS as a consequence of immoral behavior and a punishment for an undeniable sinful act. Instead of victims, these individuals were often viewed as deviants, as criminals. The stigmatization of AIDS was so strong that Patrick Buchanan, who served as Communications Director under President Reagan, wrote that the victims had "declared war upon nature, and now nature is extracting an awful retribution (AIDS)."[6] The general public was so shockingly prejudiced that records show that more than 75% of mainstream America at the time had no sympathy for those suffering and dying from AIDS.[7]

In the midst of this social and political climate, AIDS was spreading rapidly. By mid-1982, more than 450 cases had been identified, and by the end of that year, an additional 300 more cases were identified, signifying a doubling time approximately every six months! Relentless and unforgiving, the AIDS toll topped almost 16,000 by 1985, more than 8,100 of whom died from this incurable disease.[8]

## AIDS AND INTRAVENOUS DRUG USERS

IDUs are often the forgotten stepchild of the AIDS crisis, overlooked and neglected. Yet, they actually play a significant role in contributing to the global spread of AIDS. Among IDUs, HIV infection is typically spread by the sharing of contaminated needles and syringes through blood–blood transmission. To feed their craving for drugs, many IDUs use recycled contaminated syringes previously used by others because of the scarcity and high price of clean needles. According to Daniel Fernando, a street ethnographer of intravenous (IV) drug use, an addict either has to "rent a used needle or syringe either for a share of drugs or a dollar or go to a shooting gallery since he/she cannot buy and carry a needle without fear of arrest."[9]

The number of AIDS cases directly attributable to IDUs has consistently climbed annually since the epidemic began in 1981. In the United States, the relative number of drug-abusing AIDS patients soared from less than 4% in 1981 to 17% in 1984 to 28% in 1993 (see Figure 6.1).[10] By 2003, an estimated 218,000 individuals had been infected with HIV/AIDS that was directly related to their IV drug abuse. Another 93,000 cases were indirectly attributable to IV drug abuse. The disparity in the rate of IV drug abuse-associated AIDS is striking. In a survey conducted in twenty-five states, the CDC found that more than two-thirds of IV drug use-associated HIV cases were among African Americans and Hispanics.[11]

As early as 1982, concerned activists saw the inaccessibility to clean needles as a problematic impediment to preventing AIDS. Many individuals began distributing uncontaminated syringes to IDUs in hopes of saving a few lives. Doctors and nurses often left packs of syringes "in view of someone they knew who was injecting drugs, then walk[ed] out of the room."[12] The logic behind clean needle distribution was that if IV drug addicts only inject with clean needles, the probability of HIV transmission would be dramatically reduced.

In direct contrast to the U.S. experience at the time, other countries were taking a more proactive policy regarding the distribution of clean needles. The Amsterdam Junkie Union, a drug-users advocacy group, introduced the first organized NEP in the world in 1984.[13] Troubled by the actions of an inner-city pharmacist who discontinued selling syringes to IDUs, the Junkie Union, with

**Figure 6.1**
**AIDS cases attributed to intravenous drug use, 1983–1993 (CDC HIV/AIDS Surveillance Reports).**

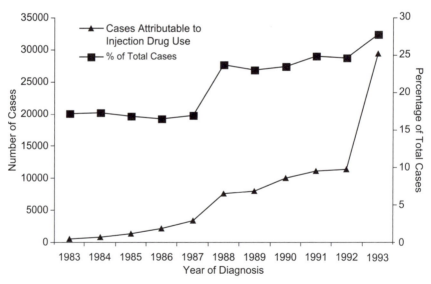

the support from the Dutch municipal Health Services, provided an anony-
mous, accessible service that became the cornerstone of HIV prevention among
IDUs. The Dutch adapted a pragmatic approach to the problem. The thinking
was that if it is not possible to cure a drug addict, then one should try to minimize the harm that the drug addict does to himself or to others.

The British followed the Dutch lead and established NEPs as a means to
reduce the spread of HIV among IDUs. A global expansion of NEPs soon followed in both developed and developing countries including Australia, Canada,
Russia, Ukraine, Bangladesh, India, and Pakistan. By 2000, at least forty-six
countries reported having at least one operating NEP in their region.[14] But not
so in the United States. The concept of NEPs had was raised in the mid-1980s,
but the program was seen by many as condoning drug use. Also at that time,
there was little proof that the program actually worked, which impeded the
proponents' arguments for establishing such programs. Almost twenty years
later, the debate is still ongoing.

## THE U.S. POLITICAL CLIMATE

From a public health perspective, needle exchange was a seemingly flawless
intervention. It addressed the identified cause and mode of transmission, and if
implemented correctly, had the potential to be 100% effective in preventing
HIV/AIDS infection. Had it been possible to ensure that every injection
involved only sterile syringes, the spread of HIV/AIDS among IDUs could
have been significantly reduced. Rational as the concept seemed, the execution
faced significant social and political obstacles in the United States.

Guided by the political agenda of the War on Drugs, the Model Drug Paraphernalia Act of 1979 (MDPA) was passed. This act made it unlawful to manufacture, sell, or distribute a wide range of devices and drug paraphernalia if it
was known that they would be used to introduce into the human body a controlled substance in violation of controlled substance laws. Many states endorsed
variants of the drug paraphernalia statutes and regulations that were closely modeled after the MDPA. Hypodermic syringes and needles were on the top of the
prohibition list. From a political perspective, NEPs were still an anathema.

From Nixon's "War on Drugs" to Nancy Reagan's "Zero Tolerance," federal
officials had consistently and vocally opposed not only the illicit use of recreational drugs, but also NEPs. As William Bennett, former director of the Office
of National Drug Control Policy under President George H.W. Bush, described,

The simple fact is that drug use is wrong ... it degrades. It makes people less than they
should be by burning way a sense of responsibility, subverting productivity, and making
a mockery of virtue. Using drugs is wrong not simply because drugs create medical
problems; it is wrong because drugs destroy one's moral sense. People addicted to drugs
neglect their duties. The lure can become so strong that soon people will do nothing
else but take drugs. They will neglect God, family, children, and jobs—everything in
life that is important, noble, and worthwhile—for the sake of drugs."[15]

The party line of the Bush I presidency was that illicit drugs were turning America into a battlefield where children were murdered and robbery was rampant. When the idea of clean needle distribution was discussed, conservatives immediately equated the distribution of clean needles with illicit drug use and feared that easier access to clean syringes might provide the impetus for more Americans to experiment with these addictive substances. Also at this time, similar sentiments were held by much of the populace.

Clean needle access also ran up against many other legal obstacles. In numerous states, syringe prescription statutes prohibited the dispensing and possession of syringes without a valid medical prescription. Some states even had statutes requiring pharmacists to obtain proof of identification from patients requesting syringes before the clean needles could be dispensed. Politics, not science, inspired these actions.

## THE TACOMA EXPERIMENT

NEP advocates knew that complete drug elimination would take time and money—two things that those fighting the AIDS epidemic did not have. In 1984, the incidence of heroin abuse reached 90,000 people, 43% greater than the incidence in 1980.[16] Yet, federal funding allocated to treating drug addiction had dramatically decreased over the years. Publicly funded treatment programs became such a rarity that among the 200,000 IV drug users in New York City, only 38,000 slots were available.[17] It was obvious that there was an urgent need to do something, even without the support of Washington.

Dave Purchase of Tacoma, Washington, took matters into his own hands. In the summer of 1988, he organized the first NEP in the United States. Originally funded by the Mahatma Kane-Jeeves Memorial Dope Fiend Trust, Dave Purchase set up a table in downtown Tacoma to exchange needles and syringes, albeit illegally. Angry community leaders and annoyed residents did everything from issuing memos to outright protesting, but like a tenacious bulldog armed with strong conviction, Purchase would not yield. Eventually, the Tacoma program expanded into the Point Defiance AIDS Project, which inspired other advocacy organizations such as the National AIDS Brigade, Act-Up, and the North American Syringe Exchange Network to launch similar efforts in other cities across the country. Perhaps not surprisingly, these programs also ran up against political and social barriers that forced the majority of them to remain underground and even operate illegally, directly defying existing laws and regulations.[18]

## THE CASE FOR HARM REDUCTION

From the perspective of Dave Purchase and other like-minded advocates, multifaceted intervention strategies were needed. That is, rather than condemning illicit drug use, programs were needed to address not only the conditions of use but also the use itself—an approach later coined as harm reduction. Why people use recreational drugs became a legitimate question that needed answers. Historically, psychologists have used four different theories to explain the etiology of substance addiction: biological, personality, behavioral, or psychosocial. The biological approach, as explained by Lovett in 1974, is built on the assumption that drug dependence results from a metabolic deficiency; addicts are inherently predisposed to drug use because genetically, they are more susceptible to severe withdrawal symptoms.[19] Personality theorists argued that there exists an "addiction-prone personality," characterized as being impulsive, egocentric, and antisocial.[20] The behaviorists opined that addiction was the byproduct of positive conditioning, that each injection provided a powerful reinforcement through an immediate rush of satisfying sensation.[21] And psychosocial modelists attempted to explain substance abuse in terms of the interaction between an individual's behavior and his environment.

Today, it is now well accepted in the social scientific community that substance abuse is caused by a complex interplay of many factors. Where a person lives, with whom he interacts, his outlook on control, his perception of goals and opportunities, as well as the availability of drugs all are important factors contributing to drug-seeking behavior. In order to rid a society of substance use, there was a need for a multidimensional approach. It would not be sufficient just to treat an addict, one also had to address the issues of poverty and homelessness, and the flow of illicit drugs from their source to the cities where they were then sold.

## THE PROHIBITIONIST REBUTTAL

From the prohibitionist perspective there is there is a thin line between morality and AIDS prevention. The thrust of NEP opposition was focused primarily on its social implications. Would we be sending a message to our children that recreational drug was condoned if we said yes to needle exchange? Would we be encouraging more illicit drug use by making clean syringes more accessible, thereby exacerbating a social sickness that was already much too prevalent? The Office of National Drug Control Policy viewed NEPs as an admission of failure. "We must not sound a retreat in the war against drugs by distributing clean needles to intravenous drug users in the hope that this will slow the spread of AIDS.... there is no getting around the fact that distributing needles facilitates drug use and undercuts the credibility of society's message that using drugs is illegal and morally wrong."[22] To the opponents, giving an intravenous drug user a needle is like handing a pyromaniac a lighter—it's irresponsible, immoral, and dangerous. In the words of General McCaffrey, director of national drug policy under President Clinton, "We owe our children an unambiguous 'no use' message ... and if they should become ensnared by drugs, we must offer them a way out, not a means to continue addictive behavior."[23]

What followed was a series of unscientific anecdotal stories in which the harmful impact of NEPs and their dangers were grossly exaggerated. Images of heroin addicts being driven to overdose and uncontrolled level of violence resonated on Capitol Hill. In the mid- to late 1980s, Congress passed a series of subsequent legislations that further prohibited federal funding of any programs that supported the distribution of new syringes. For example, Congress enacted the Mail Order Drug Paraphernalia Control Act, which was part of the Anti-Drug Abuse Act of 1986. This act provided federal enforcement with the authority to strictly prohibit the sale and transportation of drug paraphernalia, including syringes, in interstate commerce. The Department of Health and Human Services, in 1990 and 1991 appropriation acts, specifically banned the funding of NEPs unless the Surgeon General or the President of the United States could certify that such programs were effective interventions in preventing the spread of HIV without encouraging the use of illegal drugs. This action was taken before scientific findings regarding the effectiveness of NEPs even became available.

## THE SCIENTIFIC FINDINGS: WHAT DID THE RESEARCH SHOW?

Given the hostile political and economic climate that the scientific community faced in the United States, much of the early research on NEPs was conducted in Canada and Europe, where the political leadership was more receptive to clean needle access. The first sizable and systematic study assessing the effectiveness of NEPs was undertaken by a team of investigators from Middlesex Hospital and the University College London Medical School, the findings of which were published in May of 1989 in the journal *AIDS*. In this study, 121 syringe exchangers were followed for one year at which time there was a documented decrease in high-risk injection practices (i.e., the rate of lending and borrowing used needles) without any changes in the frequency of injection.[24] In another study conducted in Amsterdam, findings showed a significant reduction in needle sharing among the 263 drug users and that there was no observable rise in intravenous drug use.[25] Other studies also reported the ability of NEPs to provide protection for drug users,[26,27] to reduce the transmission rate of HIV and hepatitis C,[28,29] and to encourage enrollment into treatment programs.[30,31]

These studies, and others like them, continued to show that NEPs were associated with positive health outcomes. For example, in a comprehensive review of the effectiveness of NEPs in reducing HIV/AIDS risk behavior and HIV seroconversion among IDUs found that of the forty-two studies reviewed, twenty-eight found positive effects associated with the use of syringe exchange, two found negative associations, and fourteen found a mix of positive and negative effects.[32] Countries that introduced NEPs aggressively and early, such as Australia, had a sharp immediate decrease in IDU-associated HIV infection after implementation.[33]

Because the evidence showing that IV drug use was an important factor in HIV transmission, many prominent scientific leaders and respected organizations such as the former U.S. Surgeon General Dr. David Satcher, the Institute of Medicine, the National Institutes of Health, and the World Health Organization began giving their stamp of approval of the effectiveness of NEPs. Based on the accumulated evidence, it was clear and unequivocal that NEPs could and did save lives. In the United States, on the state and county levels, such evidence provided the impetus for some local officials to act in a positive and proactive manner. Progressive states began loosening their respective drug paraphernalia and prescription laws to permit short-term operation of NEPs albeit in limited settings. In 1987, Oregon became the first state to deregulate its drug paraphernalia law, excluding syringes from the list of paraphernalia. A total of twelve states have removed barriers from their state law to syringe access since 2003 (see Table 6.1). But on a federal level, the reaction was quite different.

As the scientific evidence accumulated, Congress and the White House continued to choose to ignore, dismiss, and dispute the scientific findings. To many of the politicians in Washington, the findings did not qualify as "proof." And for the few who conceded to scientific findings, the public endorsement of such a controversial subject was just too risky a political stance to take. Apparently, most politicians did not want to jeopardize their careers, so they stayed silent. Despite his advisory AIDS council issuing a memo, warning that the "lack of political will can no longer justify ignoring the science.... every day that goes by means more needless new infections and more human suffering," the Clinton administration did not have the courage to lift the federal funding ban; it simply was too politically risky to do otherwise.[34] Interestingly, concomitant with this subtle improvement, public opinion, too, had begun to shift to a pro harm reduction. In a 2000 survey conducted by the Lindesmith

**Table 6.1**
**Significant Events in the NEP Debate**

| Year | Significant events |
| --- | --- |
| 1979 | • Model Drug Paraphernalia Act (MDPA) was passed by the Drug Enforcement Agency: originally intended to provide a means of prosecuting operators of "head shops" |
| 1987 | • Oregon became the first state to deregulate its drug paraphernalia law to exclude syringes |
| 1984 | • Junkie Union introduced the first organized NEP in Amsterdam |
| 1988 | • Ban on federal funding for NEPs enacted; could be lifted only if the President of the United States or the Surgeon General determined that NEPs reduced the transmission of HIV infection and did not increase drug abuse |

*(Continued)*

**Table 6.1** (*Continued*)

| Year | Significant events |
|------|--------------------|
|      | • First U.S. NEP established in Tacoma, WA |
|      | • Comprehensive Alcohol Abuse, Drug Abuse, and Mental Health Amendments Act of 1988 specified that no funding could be used to "carry out any program of distributing sterile needles for the hypodermic injection of any illegal drug or distributing bleach for the purpose of cleansing needles for such hypodermic injection." |
| 1989 | • Wisconsin deregulated its drug paraphernalia law to exclude syringes |
| 1990 | • The Ryan White Comprehensive AIDS Resources Emergency Act of 1990 included provisions to prohibit funding to be spent on NEPs |
|      | • A pilot NEP was set up in New York City |
| 1992 | • Connecticut deregulated its drug paraphernalia law and prescription law |
| 1993 | • Maine deregulated its prescription law |
| 1995 | • More than 60 U.S. NEPs are in operation, in 46 cities across 21 states |
| 1997 | • Maine deregulated its drug paraphernalia law |
|      | • Minnesota deregulated its drug paraphernalia law |
| 1998 | • Secretary of the Department of Health and Human Services, Donna Shalala, issued findings required to lift the ban on federal funding, but the Clinton administration declined to seek funding for SEPs or for research |
| 2000 | • Surgeon General report endorsing NEPs as an effective means to prevent HIV was published |
|      | • New York deregulated its drug paraphernalia law and prescription law |
|      | • New Hampshire deregulated its drug paraphernalia law and prescription law |
|      | • Rhode Island deregulated its drug paraphernalia law and prescription law |
| 2001 | • Riders to the fiscal year not only prohibited the district from funding syringe exchange, but also barred a privately funded SEP from operating close to public housing and within 1,000 feet of a school |
|      | • New Mexico deregulated its drug paraphernalia law |
|      | • Hawaii deregulated its drug paraphernalia law |
| 2002 | • 2002 appropriation removed restrictions on the operation of the private SEP, but maintained the ban on federal funding |
|      | • Washington deregulated its drug paraphernalia law |
| 2003 | • Illinois deregulated its drug paraphernalia law and prescription law |
| 2005 | • At the United Nations Office on Drugs and Crime 48th Session, the commission backed away from its harm-reduction support because of political pressure from the United States |

*Source:* United Nations Office on Drugs and Crime.

Center Drug Policy Foundation, 71% of Americans surveyed express support of federal funding for NEPs.[35]

Today, four presidential administrations and five surgeon generals later, the twelve-year-old federal funding ban of NEPs continues to be in effect. The United States remains the only country in the world to directly oppose the scientifically proven cost-effective intervention in preventing HIV and AIDS. The federal ban in funding NEPs, coupled with reluctance of most politicians in Washington, DC, to take a controversial stance, left NEPs across the nation struggling. Fortunately, thanks to the very generous donations from private philanthropists, foundations, and state funding, the existing 148 NEPs in the United States were able to distribute more than 24.9 million syringes in 2005. There are some NEPs that are legally recognized now, through a patchwork of local statutory exemptions, judicial declaration, and other means that managed to circumvent existing legal restrictions. Interestingly, the number of AIDS cases that could be attributed to intravenous drug use has declined by 68% since 1994 (see Figure 6.2).

While these accomplishments represent great victories in the war against AIDS, much work remains to be done. The availability of clean syringes remains far below the estimated 1.7 billion IV drug-related injections that occur in America each year. Needle exchange in at least nineteen states is still considered illegal. Thirteen states continue to impose prescription requirement, either through statutes or regulation. Twenty-one states only permit pharmacies to sell syringes (see Table 6.2).[36] In a study conducted in 2000, over 20% of the NEPs surveyed experienced "problems with their legal status," and 30% were harassed by local law enforcement officers.[37]

**Figure 6.2**
**Number of NEPs and adult AIDS cases attributed to intravenous drug use (CDC).**

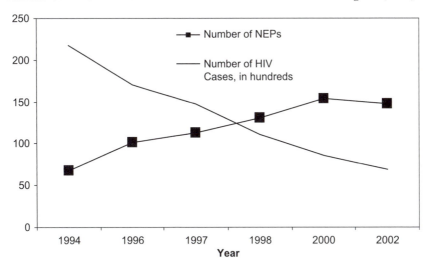

**Table 6.2**
**Needle Exchange Laws Summary, 2004**

| State | Syringe prescription requirement | Only pharmacies allowed to sell syringe | Pharmacy regulations | State drug paraphernalia law |
|-------|----------------------------------|------------------------------------------|----------------------|------------------------------|
| AL | | X | | X |
| AK | | | | None |
| AR | | | | X |
| AZ | | | | X |
| CA | X (except for use with insulin or adrenaline) | X | Record keeping, ID, display | Exempt MDs and pharmacists |
| CO | | | | Omit reference to syringes |
| CT | X (for >10 only) | X | Record keeping, display | Exempt some or all syringes |
| DC | | | | X |
| DE | X | | Record keeping, ID, display | X |
| FL | X (sale to minors only) | | | X |
| GA | | X | Information, display | Exempt pharmacists |
| HI | | | | Exempt MDs, pharmacists, and healthcare institutions |
| ID | | | | X |
| IL | X (only to minors, or for >20 only) | X | | Exempt some or all syringes |
| IN | | X | Record keeping, ID | Exempt some or all syringes |
| IA | | | | Other exemption |
| KS | | | | X |
| KY | | | Information, record keeping, ID, display | X |
| LA | | X | Information, Record keeping, ID, Display | Other exemption |

(*Continued*)

Table 6.2 (*Continued*)

| State | Syringe prescription requirement | Only pharmacies allowed to sell syringe | Pharmacy regulations | State drug paraphernalia law |
|-------|----------------------------------|-----------------------------------------|----------------------|------------------------------|
| ME | X (for >10 only) | X | ID | Exempt some or all syringes |
| MD | | X | Information, record keeping, ID | |
| MA | X | X | Record keeping, ID, display | Other exemption |
| MI | | | | Omit reference to syringes |
| MN | | X | | Exempt some or all syringes |
| MS | | | | X |
| MO | | | | X |
| MT | | | | Exempt MDs and pharmacists |
| NE | | | | X |
| NV | X (except for asthma or diabetes) | X | | Omit reference to syringes |
| NH | X (for >10 and minors only) | X | Record keeping | Exempt some or all syringes |
| NJ | X | X | Record keeping | X |
| NM | | | | Exempt pharmacists |
| NY | X (for >10 only) | X | Record keeping | Exempt some or all syringes |
| NC | | | | X |
| ND | | | | X |
| OR | | | | Exempt some or all syringes |
| OH | | X | Information, display | Exempt MDs and pharmacists |
| OK | | | | |
| PA | X | | | |
| RI | | X | Display | Exempt some or all syringes |

(*Continued*)

**Table 6.2** (*Continued*)

| State | Syringe prescription requirement | Only pharmacies allowed to sell syringe | Pharmacy regulations | State drug paraphernalia law |
|---|---|---|---|---|
| SC | | X | Information, record keeping, ID | Omit reference to syringes |
| SD | | | | |
| TN | | X | Information | Exempt MDs and pharmacists |
| TX | | | | X |
| UT | | | | X |
| VT | | | | X |
| VA | X (for minors <16 only) | X | Information, record keeping, ID, display | Other exemption |
| WA | | | Information | Exempt pharmacists |
| WV | | X | | Exempts licensees |
| WI | | | | Exempt some or all syringes |
| WY | | | | Omit reference to syringes |

*Source: Lethal Injections: The Law, Science, and Politics of Syringe Access for Injection Drug Use.*

Drug users are routinely bothered and penalized by the police while traveling to and from NEP sites, even in the "legal states." The impact of such police harassment can be tremendously damaging; it serves as barrier to discourage drug users from utilizing the invaluable services. Jamie D, a volunteer at a NEP in San Francisco, California, said in an interview with researcher Bridget Price:

Although a needle sales charge is rarely prosecuted in court, the police still use it as an arrestable offense to get people off the streets and as temporary punishment. Addicts often experience painful heroin withdrawal symptoms while in custody prior to being released by the judge. Even though the vast majority of these arrests are dismissed, the effect of them has been to increase the reluctance of injectors to carry large numbers of needles around with them. It further discourages people from coming to needle exchange and from using the services most effectively when they do come.[38]

"I think I was wrong about that," Clinton reflected at the 2002 International AIDS Conference in Barcelona, referring to his decision not to lift the federal funding ban on NEPs while in office.[39] In our fight against AIDS among IDUs, we are fortunate that a scientifically proven, cost-effective prevention strategy exists. Yet, in the United States, the usefulness of such strategy was to a large extent overshadowed by unwavering political stubbornness. The polarized debate of the pros and cons of NEPs continues to stymie federal policy. Individual states have taken action, but there is little uniformity in law among them. Some would argue that the time is long overdue to separate the War on Drugs from the War on AIDS. To do anything otherwise would be unethical, discriminatory, and irresponsible.

# —— 7 ——

# Bleak House and Beyond: How Tuberculosis Control Got Side-tracked

In the late 1980s, New York City was in the midst of a dramatic epidemic of tuberculosis (TB). With just 3% of the U.S. population, the city had 15% of the nation's TB cases. In some areas of the city, particularly the inner city, poor neighborhoods, the rate was astonishingly high. In central Harlem, for example, the incidence of TB cases was 45 times the national average![1] The resurgence of TB both in the United States and globally continues unabated. In fact, one could argue that with the increase in multidrug resistant strains of TB, the situation is far worse now than a few decades ago. What are the factors that have contributed to this situation, and could it all have been avoided with more careful attention paid to prevention and control? Has the focus on other infectious diseases eclipsed the seriousness of the TB pandemic? HIV/AIDS, for example, has dominated the headlines worldwide for so long that other equally dangerous infectious diseases have remained in the background. Were health and governmental officials too complacent in their efforts to treat those infected with TB?

The history of the rise and fall, and again rise, in TB is a sad, yet instructive one. TB is a preventable and treatable infectious disease, and there is a cost-effective cure for this disease, which is not the case for many other infectious diseases. TB is a political as much as a medical problem—and so are the solutions. It just depends on how much governments are prepared to spend. Apathy, complacency, funding cuts, and lack of access to treatment, individually and collectively, helped create the situation we face today. Ironically, unlike other deadly infectious diseases, TB more often than not responds quickly and effectively to treatment.

TB continues to pose a huge threat to global health and is today still one of the world's most serious infectious disease. More than 2 billion of the world's 6 billion people are infected with the latent form of TB (an individual has a TB infection, but does not have TB disease).[2] Whereas HIV/AIDS is estimated to kill 3 million people each year, and malaria, another prevalent potentially deadly infectious disease, kills 1 million individuals a year, TB is estimated to kill 2 million people annually.[3] "Tuberculosis is a disease that is slow and patient, relentless and effective—and year in and year out, sends millions to their graves as it travels around the globe."[4]

In 1993, 111 years after the causative organism was identified and 50 years after the introduction of effective therapy, the World Health Organization (WHO) declared TB a "global emergency." Yet, more than a decade later, this infectious disease continues to be a major killer worldwide. With millions of people traveling from country to country, and with the migration of peoples worldwide, the spread of this airborne disease, which knows no geographic boundary, is almost guaranteed. In many parts of the world, there are multidrug-resistant strains of TB now impervious to a broad menu of drugs that once effectively stopped this disease. Indeed, drug-resistant TB remains a huge and growing problem worldwide.

According to the WHO, TB infection is currently spreading at the rate of one person per second. A 1996 study by the World Bank and Harvard University reported TB as a leading cause of "healthy years lost" among men and women of reproductive age.[5] Unfortunately, a decade later, the situation has not improved. In many resource-poor countries, women bear a disproportionate burden of poverty, ill-health, malnutrition, and disease. Worldwide, for example, it is estimated that more than 900 million women are infected with TB, a disease that causes more deaths among women than all causes of maternal mortality combined. An average of fifteen years of income is lost if an individual dies of TB. One study focusing on India, where TB is endemic, found the potential for enormous social and economic disruption, which would hamper the nation's ability to develop.[6]

For those who are HIV-positive or who have full-blown AIDS, conditions that weaken the human immune system and make an individual much more vulnerable to disease, the likelihood of acquiring TB is quite high. Indeed, individuals who are HIV-positive and infected with TB are up to fifty times more likely to develop active TB than those who are HIV-negative. TB continues to be one of the leading causes of death in HIV-infected individuals as well as among other immunosuppressed IV drug users.

The history of TB control provides a cautionary tale to those entrusted to safeguard the health of the public. As history has shown, ignoring the reality that TB is a major infectious disease worldwide is dangerous; an untreated person with active TB can infect others quite easily. But history also shows that TB control programs, if poorly funded and mismanaged, can do more harm than good. Acquired resistance may develop during TB therapy because of inadequate treatment regimen, poor compliance with the treatment regimen, patients not taking the prescribed drug regimen appropriately, or treatment programs using low-quality medication.

As is the case with the other examples presented in this book, one cannot fully understand the successes and the failures of TB control without a discussion of the interaction of politics and economics. Perhaps, in this specific instance, complacency also must be mixed into the equation for a more complete understanding of how we managed to let the bacterium *Mycobacterium tuberculosis* gain the upper hand.

## WHAT IS TB?

TB, from the Greek word, *phthisis* (to waste away), is an infection caused by the bacterium *Mycobacterium tuberculosis*, which most commonly affects the lungs, but also can affect the central nervous system (meningitis), as well as the lymphatic, circulatory, genitourinary systems and bones and joints. Symptoms include a productive, prolonged cough of more than three weeks' duration, chest pain, fever, chills, and night sweats, among others. TB is spread by aerosol droplets expelled when an infected person coughs, sneezes, or spits. Those who are in close contact with an infected individual are at highest risk of becoming infected. Of note, however, is that transmission can only occur from those with *active* TB disease, not *latent* TB infections. The distinction between latent TB and active TB is important because treatment options will be different. Fortunately, most of those infected with TB have asymptomatic latent TB infection (LTBI). Indeed, not all those infected by the tubercule bacillus develop overt disease. Only a minority of cases do. The annual risk of a tuberculin-positive person developing active TB is about 0.2%.[7] Nevertheless, the pool of infected individuals worldwide is huge so even with a 0.2% conversion, millions will develop active TB each year. Among those with TB disease, history has shown that isolating those with active disease and initiating antituberculous therapy can stop the chain of transmission. Treatment with appropriate antibiotics kills the bacteria, and scar tissue eventually replaces the affected area.

## TB'S LONG HISTORY

TB is not a new disease by any stretch of the imagination. Skeletal remains indicate that prehistoric humans (4000 BC) had TB, as did ancient Egyptians, whose skeletal remains showed deformities consistent with TB disease (3000–2400 BC). Evidence of TB appears in Biblical scripture, in Chinese literature dating back to 4000 BC, and in religious books in India dating back to 2000 BC. Around 460 BC, Hippocrates identified phthisis as the most widespread disease of the time, and it was almost always fatal. Aristotle referred to phthisis and its cure around 350 BC. Although it is widely believed that

Christopher Columbus and his crew introduced TB to the New World, TB bacterium DNA was found in the mummified remains of a woman who had died in the Americas 500 years before Columbus set foot on Hispanola.

TB epidemics were frequent in Europe, reaching a peak in the late eighteenth century and early nineteenth century. In 1882, a time when TB was raging throughout Europe, the German biologist Robert Koch presented to the scientific community his discovery of the organism that caused TB. Based on the small rounded bodies (tubercles) found in diseased tissue, he coined the name tubercle bacillus. Koch received the Nobel Prize in physiology or medicine in 1905 for this discovery.

TB was made a notifiable disease in Britain after the establishment in the 1880s that the disease was contagious. There were campaigns to stop spitting in public places, and emphasis was placed on improving social conditions and educating the public about good hygiene and health habits. In their review of the history, politics, and the control of TB, Fairchild and Oppenheimer found support for the hypothesis that public health measures, along with other factors, led to falling rates of TB mortality beginning in the late nineteenth century.[8]

The TB sanatorium movement, started in Germany, advocated isolating TB-infected individuals in sanatoriums, outside of the cities, where they would purportedly benefit from fresh air, bed rest, and nutritious foods. While this movement probably helped stem the spread of the disease by removing those infected from the general public, in the early days of the movement, 75% of those who entered a sanatorium were dead within five years.

Anti-TB organizations were formed in the United States and in Europe around the end of the nineteenth century. In 1902, the first International Conference on Tuberculosis was held in Paris, and the double-barred cross (an adoption of the Cross of Lorraine used by the Knights of the First Crusade) was selected as the symbol for the fight against TB (now the symbol of the American Lung Association). In America, efforts to fund the many TB sanatoriums that were being built focused on selling Christmas seals (adapted from a method that was originated in Denmark). These seals were sold for a penny each at the post offices and thousands of dollars were raised to help children and adults with TB.

Efforts on both sides of the Atlantic Ocean were ongoing to try to find a cure or a treatment for this deadly disease, a disease of the rich and the poor. Albert Calmette and Camille Guerin, in 1906, had the first success in developing a vaccine against TB. Developed from attenuated bovine strain TB, BCG (Bacillus of Calmette and Guerin) was first used on humans in 1921 in France. To this day, many countries use the BCG vaccine as part of their TB control program, but in the United States, this vaccine is not routinely recommended now.

One of the milestones in TB history occurred in 1940 when Waksman and his team at the University of California isolated an effective anti-TB antibiotic, antinomycin.[9] While a major breakthrough, antinomycin proved to be too toxic for use in humans or animals. The development of the antibiotic streptomycin, also in the 1940s, proved to be the magic bullet. A critically ill TB patient, in 1944, was administered streptomycin, and almost immediately the bacteria disappeared from his sputum and he made a rapid recovery. *M. tuberculosis* met its match. A rapid succession of drugs helped make treatment a reality. But, prevention and control of TB was, and still is, a pressing public health issue.

## TB PREVENTION AND CONTROL IN THE UNITED STATES

TB prevention and control efforts tended to focus on three strategies: (1) identify and treat those with TB, (2) find and evaluate individuals who have been in contact with TB patients to determine whether they have TB infection or disease, and if so, then treat them and make sure that they complete the course of therapy, and (3) test high-risk groups for TB infection. This strategy has not changed much over the decades. In the late nineteenth century in New York City, for example, Dr. Hermann Michael Biggs, the Chief Inspector of the Division of Pathology, Bacteriology, and Disinfection for the New York City Board of Health, made similar recommendations to the Board of Health. The key, then and now, is to find those individuals with active TB and treat them. An educational campaign to alert the public of the dangers that the disease posses to himself/herself and to others should accompany any treatment and control program.

While Dr Biggs was a pioneer in the development of a model TB control program that was emulated by other health departments across the country, the federal government's control program did not occur until the mid-1940s when the 1944 Public Health Service Act (Public Law 78-410) authorized the establishment of a TB control program (Tuberculosis Control Division in the Bureau of State Services of the Public Health Service). The Public Health Service provided supplemental fiscal support to state and local health departments for TB control activities through formula grants and special grants-in-aid. The focus was to be on case finding as well as measures for prevention, treatment, and control.

Mass x-ray screening for TB was organized in 1947, and over 20 million individuals were screened. Well-known figures posing for an x-ray, Santa Claus being one such example, were used in advertisements to encourage the public to be screened. With the introduction of antibiotic drugs to treat TB in the late 1940s and early 1950s, a new era in TB control was introduced. TB patients were treated in hospitals and local community clinics rather than sanatoriums. Morbidity declined dramatically. By 1970, only a few sanatoriums and TB hospitals remained.

Declining TB mortality, however, resulted in a shortsighted cutback in funding from federal, state, and local agencies responsible for TB control. Since the incidence and prevalence of TB was low, money that had been allocated to TB programs was allocated to fund other programs. Unfortunately, a series of cumulative events created a situation that caught officials off-guard. The public health infrastructure that had so successfully addressed TB treatment, control, and prevention was not prepared for what was to come.

In 1989, the Centers for Disease Control and Prevention (CDC), the U.S. federal government's lead agency for TB prevention, control, and elimination, published *A Strategic Plan for the Elimination of Tuberculosis in the United States*.[10] Building on the success of past TB detection and control programs, the plan was to eliminate TB in the United States by 2010. Several events collided to make it almost impossible to achieve this objective. In particular, HIV/AIDS, first identified around this time, had a direct impact on the renewed rise of TB. In hindsight, we now know that TB and HIV coinfections strained the health system, and to make matters more complicated, multidrug-resistant TB was confounding treatment and control efforts. Mortality was on the increase, and there was a serious need to develop new TB control programs to address this issue.

Concomitant with the HIV/AIDS epidemic and its effect on the TB rate, other factors also contributed to the renewed rise in the incidence of TB. Nearly half of the reported new cases of TB were occurring in individuals who immigrated to the United States. These foreign-born individuals came from countries where TB is endemic (Mexico, the Philippines, China, India, and Vietnam). Indeed, the elimination of TB was (and still is) seriously threatened by the very high rates among foreign-born individuals who migrated to other areas. The TB case rate among foreign-born persons is at least eight times higher than among U.S.-born individuals.[11]

During the 1980s, TB was making a menacing comeback; the incidence increased an alarming 20% from 1985 to 1992.[12] In hindsight, the resurgence can be linked to the significant government funding cutbacks for TB during the 1970s. The funding cutbacks that were put in place resulted in the deterioration of existing TB control programs, and the end result was that TB control officials had very few resources with which to address the resurgence of the disease. Also, those receiving treatment, many of whom who used injection drugs or had psychiatric problems, did not take their medicines regularly. This situation allowed patients with infectious TB to remain a threat to others; relapse was frequent. Worst of all, noncompliance led to the emergence of drug-resistant cases of TB.

The CDC reacted to the situation by publishing the National Action Plan to Combat Multidrug-Resistant Tuberculosis in 1992 to complement the 1989 TB elimination document.[13] In an effort to highlight the "cycle of neglect," which was coined to characterize TB control efforts, the CDC also commissioned the Institute of Medicine (IOM) to conduct a study to determine whether TB elimination was still feasible as a national goal, and if so, to provide recommendations on how to make that goal a reality. The report, *Ending Neglect: The Elimination of Tuberculosis in the United States*, concluded that TB elimination was feasible but would require "aggressive and decisive action beyond what is now in effect."[14] The IOM called for controlling TB; developing new tools for TB diagnosis, treatment, and prevention; increasing the U.S. effort to fight the global epidemic; and mobilizing and sustaining public support for TB elimination. A new tough-love approach, including forcible detention, was advocated.

There actually was a decline in the incidence of TB during the 1990s, which can be directly attributable to the increase in treatment and control activities. From 1992 to 2001, for example, the incidence of TB in the United States decreased by 40%.[15] Again, this dramatic reduction is attributed to effective TB control programs that identified people with TB, prompt initiation of appropriate therapy, and innovative efforts to ensure that therapy would be completed. But, the decline in rates was not uniform.

One study that looked at factors associated with decreases in TB cases in the United States from 1993 and 1994 found that the decrease was confined to U.S.-born individuals primarily as a direct result of treatment and control activities. The researchers cautioned that continued success in preventing the occurrence of active TB would require sustained efforts to ensure appropriate treatment and control for all infected persons.[16]

While treatment and control efforts were benefiting U.S.-born individuals, TB remained a serious public health problem among certain population groups; that is, foreign-born persons, those in correctional facilities, the homeless, those with HIV/AIDS, and drug abusers.[17] Reducing the large reservoir of individuals at risk for progression to active TB, however, is a daunting task. And without adequate funding, the job is even harder.

## THE GLOBAL EMERGENCY OF TB

To control TB in the United States, global control is necessary. That is, well-organized and well-funded control programs are needed to address the epidemic at the source, which refers primarily to resource-poor countries. Over the past decade, twenty-the countries accounted for 80% of all new TB cases, with more than half concentrated in five countries (Bangladesh, China, India, Indonesia, and Nigeria).[18] Given that disease surveillance is rudimentary in these countries, surveys of TB prevalence, based on case-finding and bacteriological surveys, are notoriously unreliable. The estimated total number of cases is most probably an underestimate of the true number of cases.

The Global Partnership to Stop TB is a worldwide movement whose objective is to accelerate social and political action to stop the spread of TB.[19] The Stop TB mission is to ensure that every TB patient has access to TB treatment; to protect vulnerable populations from acquiring TB; and to reduce the social and economic toll that TB exacts from families, communities, and nations. The Partnership's approach is coordinated and multinational. But, as the history of TB clearly shows, money is needed to effectively eliminate TB worldwide. These efforts were given a significant boost when Bill and Melinda Gates announced in 2006 that their charitable foundation would triple its funding from $300 million to $900 million for TB eradication.[20]

## HOW TO EFFECT TB CONTROL: "DOT"

The goals of anti-TB therapy include ensuring a cure without relapse, preventing death, stopping transmission of *M. tuberculosis*, and preventing the emergence of drug-resistant disease.[21] In the United States, for example, state and local health departments have legal responsibility for the prevention and control of TB. Identifying persons who have TB, ensuring that they complete appropriate therapy, conducting outreach to find and screen individuals who have been in contact with TB patients to determine whether they too have TB infection or disease and then provide them with appropriate treatment, and screening high-risk populations to detect those who are infected with *M. tuberculosis* and who would benefit from therapy to prevent the infection from progressing to TB disease.

Successful treatment of TB depends on prescribing an appropriate drug regimen, as well as ensuring that treatment is completed. Naturally, patient compliance is a key factor in treatment success. Evidence clearly shows that self-administered therapy is not very effective primarily because a significant proportion of patients receiving self-administered treatment do not adhere to treatment and stop before completing the full course as prescribed.[22] Those treatment and control programs that provide medications directly to the person and have a medical or public health professional actually watch the individual swallow the drugs (directly observed therapy—DOT) have been shown to be very effective. Indeed, DOT has been lauded as the key to recent successes of the American TB-control efforts, as well as for other nations, and this method is now the internationally recommended approach to TB control.

There are five components to DOT: (1) political commitment to sustained TB control, (2) access to TB sputum microscopy, (3) standardized short-course chemotherapy, (4) uninterrupted supply of drugs, and (5) a standardized recording and reporting system enabling assessment of outcome in all patients. A new variation on DOT has been designed recently: directly observed treatment, short-course, or DOTS. DOTS is similar to DOT in that an observer watches and helps the patient swallow the tablets for the entire short course of treatment. In a sense, DOT is one element of the DOTS strategy. Standard short-course regimens can cure more than 90% of new, drug-susceptible TB cases.[23] DOTS, too, has become the internationally recommended approach to TB control, with its focus on case detection and treatment success and three measures of impact (incidence, prevalence, and mortality reduction).

As of the year 2000, 149 countries had adopted the DOTS strategy. Both DOT and DOTS have helped ensure a higher completion rate, helped prevent the emergence of drug-resistant TB, and enhanced TB control by reducing transmission of tubercule bacilli as well as the emergence of drug-resistant strains.[24] In areas where DOTS was implemented, cure rates of up to 95% were recorded; the DOTS strategy was ranked by the World Bank as one of the most cost-effective of all health interventions.[25] More than 17 million TB patients have been treated in DOTS programs around the world between 1994 and 2003.

## THE NEW GLOBAL CHALLENGE: MULTIDRUG-RESISTANT TB AND EXTREME MULTIDRUG-RESISTANT TB

We now know that TB control programs that are underfunded often do more harm than good. Point in fact, inadequate TB control now appears to be a major cause of MDR-TB. MDR-TB is a form of TB that is resistant to two or more of the primary drugs used for the treatment of TB, primarily isoniazid and rifampicin. Resistance to one or several forms of treatment occurs when the bacteria develops the ability to withstand antibiotic attack and relays that ability to newly produced bacteria. Resistance to anti-TB drugs in populations is a phenomenon that occurs primarily because of poorly managed TB care. Problems include incorrect drug-prescribing practices by providers, poor-quality drugs or erratic supply of drugs, and also patient nonadherence.

The WHO estimates that up to 50 million persons worldwide may be infected with drug-resistant strains of TB. It is estimated that 300,000 new cases of MDR-TB are diagnosed around the world each year, and 79% of the MDR-TB cases now show resistance to three or more drugs.[26] Sadly, mortality rates of MDR-TB are comparable with those for TB in the days before the availability of antibiotics. The HIV/AIDS epidemic has most certainly complicated the ability to gain an upper hand in the battle to eradicate TB. Multidrug-resistant strains of TB have been a particular concern among HIV-infected individuals. Clearly, the success of treatment depends on how quickly a case of TB is identified as drug resistant and whether an effective drug therapy is available. Unfortunately, the second-line drugs used in cases of MDR-TB are often less effective and more likely to cause side effects.[27] Compounding the difficulties of dealing with this new wrinkle in TB control, it is well known that multidrug-resistant strains of TB are not only more difficult to treat, but they are also more costly; one case of MDR-TB is estimated to cost up to $250,000 to treat.[28] Moreover, the case fatality is extremely high because the overwhelming majority of those with MDR-TB die relatively quickly.

While MDR-TB is certainly alarming, very recently a new and extremely dangerous form of TB was identified: a "virtually untreatable" form of TB has now emerged according to WHO. Extreme drug-resistant TB (XDR-TB), has been seen worldwide, including the United States, Eastern Europe, and Africa. XDR-TB, in addition to the two first-line drugs used to treat TB, is also resistant to three or more of the six classes of second-line drugs. What makes this strain of TB so lethal is that XDR-TB can infect even the healthiest of people. While the chance of survival is greater among healthy people because these individuals are more likely to be able to fight off the disease, those who have compromised immune systems due to HIV and AIDS who develop XDR-TB usually will die within a month. In the most recent outbreak of XDR-TB located in Kwazulu-Natal, in South Africa, fifty-three patients were found with XDR-TB. Of these, fifty-two died within twenty-five days, and forty-four of the fifty-three were tested for HIV and found to be HIV positive. Some experts think that this is just the "tip of the iceberg." Since South Africa is the epicenter of HIV and TB, both of these infectious diseases have the capacity to fast-track MDR into an uncontrollable XDR-TB epidemic. If this epidemic gets out of control, the impact on a regional and global basis could be severe. XDR-TB could have a bigger impact on developing nations, especially Africa, because of the very high prevalence of HIV and AIDS.

WHO has expressed concern over the emergence of the virulent drug-resistant strains of TB and is calling for measures to be strengthened and implemented to prevent the global spread of the deadly extreme TB strains. Globally, there have been just 347 identified cases of XDR-TB, mainly in the former Soviet Union and in Asia, but the emergence of XDR-TB anywhere in the world poses a threat everywhere in the world. Paul Sommerfeld of TB Alert said that XDR-TB is very serious. For the world as a whole, it is potentially extremely worrying that this kind of resistance is appearing. We are potentially getting close to a bacterium that we have no tools, no weapons against. This form of TB is a likely death sentence.

## WHAT HAVE WE LEARNED?

TB is as much a social and political disease as it is a medical one. Globally, TB is preventable and treatable, but it all depends on how much each government is willing and able to spend to stem the epidemic. Without adequate surveillance methods, with delays in detecting infected individuals, and without improving treatment compliance, it is a sure bet that the situation will get much worse. We know from past experience that failure to ensure treatment compliance and cutbacks in funding are the main causes of the epidemic of MDR-TB. If nothing changes, if we do not strengthen and expand detection and treatment programs, it is estimated that by 2020, nearly 1 billion additional individuals will be newly infected with TB, 200 million will become sick, and 35 million will die. The WHO Chairman of Mycobacterial Diseases Therapy, Jacques Grosset, said over a decade ago: "because the problems are political, not medical, the solution is political. . . ."[29]

# — 8 —

## Science, Politics, and the Regulation of Dietary Supplements

When the Baltimore Orioles pitcher, Steve Bechler, died of heatstroke in 2003, ephedra, a dietary supplement, was suspected as a contributing factor in his death. Ephedra, a derivative of the Chinese herb Ma huang was used by many people to help in weight loss, to boost energy, and to enhance sports performance. Its synthetic version, ephedrine, is used as a treatment for colds and asthma and is categorized as a drug. As such, *ephedrine* is regulated by the Food and Drug Administration (FDA). *Ephedra*, however, is categorized as a dietary supplement and is exempt from federal regulation. As Bechler's tragic death clearly showed, there are serious adverse effects associated with this herbal product, including its powerful stimulatory effects on the cardiovascular and central nervous systems.

While perhaps a dramatic way to shed light on the hidden dangers of many dietary supplements and herbal products currently widely available, the fact remains that these products, ranging from vitamins, minerals, herbs, amino acids, and enzymes, are available without prescription and, because they are not considered medicines, are not required to undergo the rigorous testing that drugs do before they go on the market. There is strong evidence that some dietary supplements can cause serious adverse reactions, including injury and even death. Since less than 1% of serious adverse events are reported to the FDA, the true magnitude of how many people experience an adverse reaction (mild, moderate, or serious) linked to a dietary supplement is really not known. In America, dietary supplements are considered safe until proven dangerous, whereas drugs are dangerous until proven safe.

For years the FDA has struggled to formulate an effective regulatory approach for dietary supplements but has been seriously hampered by existing federal law, which clearly states that dietary supplements are to be regulated like foods instead of drugs. While the manufacturers of dietary supplements are responsible for ensuring that their products are safe and that their label claims are accurate and truthful, by law, they are not *required* to conduct studies to show a supplement's safety before the product is marketed nor do they have to prove that their product is effective. Of course, many dietary supplements, especially some vitamins and minerals, have been shown to be safe and even beneficial, especially when people take the recommended amount/dose of the product. But many other dietary supplement products have neither been shown to be effective nor safe. Listing the word "natural" on the box does not always mean "safe." Indeed, just because the word "natural" is on the bottle or box does not always mean that the product is "without harmful effects."

Many supplements contain active ingredients that can have strong effects in the body. In fact, taking a combination of supplements, using these products together with prescription medicine, or substituting them in place of prescribed medicines could lead to harmful or even life-threatening results. Also, more is not necessarily better. Some products can be harmful when consumed in high amounts; vitamin A is an excellent example of a product that is harmful when taken in large amounts. Nevertheless, the majority of consumers taking dietary supplements believe that these products are either reasonably or completely safe. Dietary supplement advocates correctly point out that far more people experience adverse events from prescription drugs. But, because the law does not require the reporting of adverse events for dietary supplements, the lack of data may be masking a potentially serious situation.

The dietary supplement industry would have the public believe that supplements can help stave off disease, improve one's energy level, and that they are safe. In some cases, their claims are correct. In other cases, the epidemiological evidence is not as clearcut or as positive. Given that so many people consume one or more dietary supplements on a regular basis, there are growing concerns about the efficacy and safety of these products, which are readily and easily available for purchase over-the-counter in supermarkets, drug stores, health food stores, and on the Internet. Former FDA Commissioner, Dr. Mark B. McClellan, characterized the situation well when he was quoted in an AARP (American Association of Retired Persons) Bulletin as saying that it is a "buyer beware market."[1] Ensuring dietary supplement product safety, standards, and oversight remain a challenge given the restraints and drawbacks to the system of surveillance of these products.

This chapter reviews the science and the politics of the regulation of dietary supplements, and it will be shown that the stakes are high for both the consumer as well as the manufacturer.

## WHAT IS A DIETARY SUPPLEMENT?

Dietary supplements are intended to supplement the diet. Congress defined the term "dietary supplement" in the Dietary Supplement Health and Education

Act (DSHEA) of 1994 to refer to a product taken by mouth that contains a "dietary ingredient" intended to supplement the diet.[2] The "dietary ingredients" in these products may include: vitamins, minerals, herbs or other botanicals, amino acids, and substances such as enzymes, organ tissues, glandulars, and metabolites.

*Vitamins* are chemicals that cannot be made by the body but are necessary for certain functions. Vitamins are essential nutrients for the healthy maintenance of the cells, tissues, and organs that make up a multicellular organism; they also enable a multicellular life-form to efficiently use chemical energy provided by food eaten, and to help process the proteins, carbohydrates, and fats required for respiration. For example, vitamin C is important for the construction of strong connective tissue, and vitamin D is important for healthy bones. In humans there are thirteen vitamins, divided into two groups; four fat-soluble vitamins (A, D, E, and K), and nine water-soluble vitamins (eight B vitamins and vitamin C).

*Minerals* are essential elements, which are required in trace amounts for normal body function. Minerals provide the spark for many of the body's cellular processes and keep them running efficiently. Without these finely tuned chemical reactions, no organism could function. They are necessary in processes such as the action of enzyme systems, the contraction of muscles, nerve reactions, and the clotting of blood. Calcium, magnesium, sodium, potassium, and chloride, for example, are important minerals necessary for health and well-being.

*Herbal supplements* are generally defined as any form of a plant or plant product and contain complicated mixtures of organic chemicals, the levels of which may vary substantially depending upon many factors related to the growth, production, and processing of the herbal product.[3] Herbal products may contain a single herb or combinations of several different herbs believed to have complementary effects. Some herbal products, including many traditional Chinese medicines, also may include animal products and minerals. Ginkgo biloba, saw palmetto, and St. John's wort are examples of commonly used herbals (see Table 8.1 for a listing of the ten most commonly used herbal products in the United States).

*Amino acids* are the building blocks of protein. Twenty amino acids are needed to build the various proteins used in the growth, repair, and maintenance of body tissues. Eleven of these amino acids can be made by the body itself, while the other nine (called essential amino acids) must come from the diet. Foods of animal origin, such as meat and poultry, fish, eggs, and dairy products, are the richest dietary sources of the essential amino acids. The vast majority of Americans eat more than enough protein and also more than enough of each essential amino acid for normal purposes.

Dietary supplements products can be extracts or concentrates and may be found in many forms such as tablets, capsules, softgels, gelcaps, liquids, or powders. They can also be in other forms, such as a bar; but, whatever the form, information on the label must not represent the product as a conventional food or a sole item of a meal or diet. To ensure a dietary supplement product's

**Table 8.1**
**Ten Most Commonly Used Herbs in the United States**

| Herb | Common use |
|------|-----------|
| 1. Echinacea | Upper respiratory tract infection |
| 2. Garlic | Hypercholesterolemia |
| 3. Ginkgo biloba | Dementia, cognitive impairment |
| 4. Saw palmetto | Benign prostatic hyperplasia |
| 5. Ginseng | Physical performance |
| 6. Grape seed extract | Venous insufficiency |
| 7. Green tea | Cancer |
| 8. St. John's wort | Depression |
| 9. Bilberry | Vision impairment |
| 10. Aloe | Wound healing/dermatitis |

*Source:* Bent, S., and Ko, R. Commonly used herbal medicines in the United States: A review. *Am J Med.* 2004;116:478–485.

status as a dietary supplement, the label must be consistent with the statutes inherent in the DSHEA. Further discussion of the DSHEA follows later in the chapter.

## WHO TAKES DIETARY SUPPLEMENTS?

The use of dietary supplements in the United States has increased dramatically during the last decade. A 1990 survey on supplement use, for example, documented a 12-month prevalence of 2.5% for use of any herbal preparation.[4] When a similar survey was conducted in 1997, the prevalence increased to 12%, demonstrating a rather large increase in the use of these substances over a relatively short period of time.[5] More recent findings estimate that one-fifth of the American population currently uses at least one type of dietary supplement daily.[6] Of course, use differs by product (vitamin, herbal, etc.), age of user, and gender, but the numbers clearly indicate that a lot of people are using a lot of different products every day.[7] Not surprisingly, the dietary supplement industry is huge; sales in 2006 in the United States were estimated to be $20 billion. There are over 1,000 manufacturers marketing 29,000 products, with an average of 1,000 new products developed each year.[8]

Why do people consume dietary supplements? Based on results of multiple national opinion surveys, the most common reasons for consuming dietary supplements are to supplement the diet with vitamins and minerals and to help in the treatment of medical conditions (arthritis, depression, colds, and cancer).[9] In one survey, over one-third of the respondents said that they take vitamins/

mineral supplements because they feel it is healthy and/or good for them, and 16% said that they take herbals because they feel these products are healthy and/or good for them.[10] Many users feel so strongly about the potential health benefits of some of the products that they would continue to take the supplements even if they were shown to be ineffective in scientifically conducted clinical studies! Most of those who consume dietary supplements take two or more supplements a day, and the majority do not discuss the use of dietary supplements with their doctors because they believe that the physicians know little or nothing about these products and may be biased against them.

## EFFICACY OF DIETARY SUPPLEMENTS

For years, millions of Americans have spent billions of dollars on alternative remedies whose benefits and risks have not been rigorously studied. Supplements are often perceived as safe because they are "natural," but what the public needs to understand is that many dietary supplements can and do have a powerful effect on the body. Vitamin excess is indeed possible with supplementation, particularly for fat-soluble vitamins such as vitamin A and vitamin K. As such, there are legitimate concerns about the safety of taking dietary supplements. Many supplements have been associated with adverse events that include all levels of severity and organ systems.[11] The "naturalness" of herbals and vitamins is not a guarantee that the product will not produce an adverse event. Potential adverse events have been noted ranging from mild (allergic reactions, nausea, and diarrhea) to quite serious (high blood pressure, elevated heart rate, stroke, and liver dysfunction). Ginkgo biloba and vitamin E, for example, can decrease blood clotting, which may be beneficial for individuals with vascular disease but disastrous for people who are already taking blood thinners (including aspirin) or who are scheduled to undergo surgery.

Herbals, in particular, contain potent bioactive substances, and many dangerous and lethal side effects have been reported from the use of some herbal products.[12] For example, St. John's wort can increase the effects of prescription drugs used to treat depression and can also interfere with drugs used to treat HIV infection and cancer. Ginseng can increase the stimulant effects of caffeine and can lower blood sugar levels, thus possibly interfering with prescription drugs prescribed for diabetes. There have been numerous reports about cardiovascular and central nervous system risks of dietary supplements rich in ephedra alkaloids.[13] Ephedra was finally banned by the FDA because of the serious adverse effects seen in those taking products containing this herbal.

Research to assess the safety, efficacy, and effectiveness of dietary supplements is being conducted with the National Center for Complementary and Alternative Medicine, a division of the National Institutes of Health, funding most of the studies. Such information is important to help the consumer better understand and figure out which products and supplements are safe and which

are worth taking. Results from studies that have looked at the health benefits of
many supplements findings, however, have been mixed (depending on the supplement under study) in some cases, and quite clear in other instances, again
depending on the supplement. The paucity of clinical trials (double-blind,
placebo-controlled), however, makes it difficult to truly assess a supplement's
benefits and risks. (An excellent source for systematic reviews and meta-analyses
of clinical trials published on dietary supplement safety and efficacy can be
found by accessing the Cochrane Library at www.cochrane.org/reviews). The
Institute of Medicine also has issued a report on the safety and efficacy of dietary supplements entitled, *Dietary Supplements: A Framework for Evaluating
Safety* (www.iom.org).

The following is not meant to be an exhaustive listing of the voluminous
literature on the subject. Sometimes separating out the myth from the reality is
not so easy. A large part of the problem is the difficulty in designing a rigorous
study. It must be acknowledged that the evidence for the safety and efficacy of
commonly used herbs and supplements is limited, and of those studies that
have been conducted, methodological flaws in study design make it difficult to
ascertain a product's effectiveness, risks, and benefits. Also, variations in the
product (lack of standardization) and outcome assessment make it hard to
definitively determine a product's efficacy.

**The claim:** Vitamin E will help prevent heart disease and cancer.

**The reality:** Vitamin E is fat soluble and has antioxidant properties. Like
other antioxidants, vitamin E was thought to have the ability to prevent
diseases, in particular, atherosclerotic disease. Vitamin E was hailed as a wonder vitamin in the early 1990s after two large survey studies reported that male
and female health professionals who said that they took a supplement of up to
400 IU every day had fewer reports of heart disease and cancer than their peers
who did not take the supplement.[14,15] In these prospective, observational studies involving individuals without known cardiovascular disease, the use of
vitamin E supplements (400 IU per day) had been associated with a 20%–40%
reduction in the risk of coronary disease.[16] Primarily because of the positive
findings of this study, by the year 2000, an estimated 23 million people were
taking vitamin E. Follow-up double-blind, placebo-controlled studies, however,
could not substantiate these findings.

To test whether vitamin E supplementation decreases risks of cardiovascular
disease and cancer among healthy women, almost 40,000 women aged at least
45 years were randomly assigned to receive vitamin E (600 IU taken every
other day) or placebo and aspirin or placebo. The data from this large trial
found that vitamin E provided no overall benefit for major cardiovascular
events or cancer nor did it decrease the cardiovascular mortality in healthy
women.[17] The researchers concluded that the data did not support recommending vitamin E supplementation for cardiovascular disease or cancer prevention
among healthy women. A review of other clinical trials designed to evaluate
the safety and efficacy of vitamin E supplementation in cardiovascular disease

and cancer prevention did not find a protective benefit of vitamin E for either heart disease or for cancer.[18]

Vitamin E was also thought to help protect the brain from Alzheimer's disease, but a large placebo-controlled study found that a high daily dose of the vitamin did not slow mild cognitive impairment.[19] Specifically, subjects with mild cognitive impairment were randomly assigned to receive 2000 IU of vitamin E daily, 10 mg of donepezil, or placebo for three years. There were no significant differences in the probability of progression to Alzheimer's disease in the vitamin E group; vitamin E had no benefit in patients with mild cognitive impairment.

It was also hypothesized that vitamin E supplementation could reduce the risk of cancer. Several large clinical trials showed no benefit in terms of reducing the risk of breast cancer,[20] and the reduction in the risk of colon cancer was mixed.[21] On the positive side, there is scant evidence that vitamin E is harmful. Hence, many continue to take a daily capsule of vitamin E "just in case" there might be some positive effect yet to be documented.

**The claim:** Taking beta-carotene can help prevent cancer.

**The reality:** Carotenoids are a class of yellow, orange, and red plant-derived compounds. Interest in carotenoids, especially beta-carotene, initially arose because it was thought that their antioxidant effects could prevent cardiovascular disease and cancer. The antioxidant beta-carotene, in particular, was thought to prevent cancer-causing substances from damaging DNA. Observational studies found a protective effect of beta-carotene intake and lung cancer, but large-scale, placebo-controlled, randomized, controlled trials could not corroborate these findings. Two large National Cancer Institute-funded chemoprevention trials were conducted on thousands of individuals who were considered to be at high risk for developing lung cancer. The purpose of these trials was to ascertain whether certain vitamin supplements would prevent lung and other cancers. After years of follow up on thousands of individuals, neither the Beta Carotene and Retinol Efficacy Trial (CARET) nor the Alpha-Tocopherol, Beta Carotene Cancer Prevention Trial showed a benefit from taking this supplement.[22] In fact, among smokers, beta-carotene supplementation actually increased the risk of lung cancer. The increased risks for lung cancer that occurred in participants supplemented with beta-carotene began to fall soon after the individuals stopped taking the vitamin, and were similar to the placebo group within four years. The conclusion was that beta-carotene supplementation should be avoided by smokers, in particular. Further, at least five randomized trials have shown no reduction in colorectal cancer risk with beta-carotene supplementation[23–27], and no benefit has been found in terms of the risk reduction of breast cancer.[28]

**The claim:** Vitamin B supplementation can prevent heart attacks and strokes.

**The reality:** It was widely accepted that B vitamins (folic acid, vitamin B12, and vitamin B6) are protective against homocysteine, an amino acid that is a risk factor for heart disease. Homocysteine was hypothesized to affect atherosclerotic processes. Elevated plasma total homocysteine level is a major risk factor for coronary disease. Folic acid and vitamins B6 and B12 are important regulators of the metabolism of homocysteine in the body. Medical studies, however, showed that this vitamin therapy was really not effective, especially among those with pre-existing cardiovascular disease.

A meta-analysis of randomized, controlled trials was conducted to evaluate the effects of folic acid supplementation on risk of cardiovascular diseases and all-cause mortality among individuals with pre-existing cardiovascular or renal disease. Findings showed that folic acid supplementation did not reduce the risk of cardiovascular diseases or all-cause mortality in this trial.[29] Further, another trial designed to assess whether supplementation of folic acid and B vitamins would reduce the risk of major cardiovascular events in patients with vascular disease did not find that supplementation reduced the risk in these individuals.[30] That is, the group taking the vitamin supplement therapy had a similar number of heart attacks and strokes as did the group taking the placebo. Consistent results from several large studies led to the unequivocal conclusion that there is no clinical benefit in taking folic acid and vitamin B12 (with without vitamin B6) in patients with established vascular disease.

It was also hypothesized that higher dietary folate intake could reduce the risk of colon and breast cancer. The evidence, however, is not based on randomized trials, thus making it difficult to draw reliable conclusions about the benefits of folate supplementation for this purpose.

**The claim:** Glucosamine and chondroitin sulfate alleviate arthritis pain.

**The reality:** Two widely used nutritional supplements made from animal cartilage and shellfish, glucosamine and chondroitin sulfate, were widely touted as being effective means for alleviating osteoarthritis pain. These products generated $1.7 billion in sales in 2005 despite any evidence that they actually did any good. In a large-scale clinical study, meant to provide quantifiable evidence of the effectiveness of these supplements, findings showed no effect for glucosamine, chondroitin, or a combination of the two. That is, the supplements turned out to be no better than the placebo in relieving mild arthritis pain.[31] While the studies did not find statistically significant benefits, there was no real harm either. Maybe there was a placebo effect (just because you are taking a pill that you think can help you makes you think that there is a benefit), or maybe the study population was not representative of the general population with mild arthritis. Despite the epidemiologic evidence, many arthritis patients swear by the supplements. Those who insist that the treatments work for them were not swayed by the findings.

**The claim:** Echinacea will prevent you from getting a cold.

**The reality:** Echinacea was one of the most commonly used herbal remedies in the United States with reported sales in the hundreds of million dollars annually. There have been several clinical trials conducted, which suggested that Echinacea may be an efficacious treatment for upper respiratory tract infections, but methodological flaws in these studies are believed to have compromised the findings. That is, variations in quality and design of the studies make it difficult to state with certainty that Echinacea is effective in preventing one from developing a cold. Two better designed studies found no benefit at all in taking Echinacea to ward off a cold.[32,33] A study looking at the efficacy and safety of Echinacea in treating upper respiratory tract infections in children also found no benefit in treating upper respiratory tract symptoms in patients aged 2 to 11 years old, and its use was associated with an increased risk of rash.[34] Even though studies could not show a statistical benefit in preventing or treating colds with Echinacea, many individuals continue to take this supplement in hopes of either preventing a cold or mitigating the symptoms. Since there are no serious side effects from this product, the downside risks of taking Echinacea are quite low.

**The claim:** St. John's wort is beneficial in the treatment of depression.

**The reality:** St. John's wort has been studied extensively as a means of treating depression. The active ingredients, hypericin and hyperforin, inhibit the reuptake of monoamines, including serotonin, noradrenaline, and dopamine. Several systematic reviews all concluded that the herb is beneficial in the treatment of depression[35–37] One study comparing St. John's wort with the tricyclic antidepressant, Imiprimine, found the herb to be more effective with fewer reported side effects.[38] And, two randomized, controlled trials conducted in the United States found that the herb was not effective in *major* depression but more so in *mild to moderate* forms of the disease.[39,40]

Concern has been raised about adverse interactions of St. John's wort with some prescription drugs, and the fact that many individuals take this herb without telling their physician could pose a problem. Further, there is a risk that people with clinical depression may self-medicate with St. John's wort rather than seek care from a therapist and receive an anti-depressant.

**The claim:** DHEA supplements are rejuvenating anti-aging agents.

**The reality:** Levels of the adrenal sex steroid dehydroepiandrosterone (DHEA) fall progressively after age thirty. DHEA, a steroid that is a precursor to the sex hormones testosterone and estrogen, has been marketed as the "foundation of youth" hormone and as a rejuvenating agent. In the United States, sales of the supplement topped $50 million in 2005. Some athletes use DHEA and testosterone to try to boost performance. Researchers, however, wondered if DHEA could help older people improve their strength and physical performance and fight diabetes and heart disease.

In recent years, several randomized, placebo-controlled trials looked at the efficacy of DHEA in older adults. The conclusion drawn from the findings of these trials was that DHEA showed no effect on body composition, physical performance, or insulin sensitivity compared with placebo.[41,42] Basically, there is no evidence that this supplement can or did stop the aging process or improve strength or physical performance. Although not the elixir of youth, there were no adverse events reported among those taking DHEA.

In summary, the epidemiologic evidence belies the reports of misleading labeling, as well as false claims about many dietary supplement products, making it more urgent to press for more stringent regulation of herbals and other supplements. Consumers may be misled by a manufacturer's claim that its product can treat, prevent, or cure specific diseases when in fact there is no such supporting evidence. Despite these concerns, not all supplements are unsafe. Some have been shown to confer proven benefits and are accurately labeled. Systematic reviews, for example, have found statistically significant benefits of garlic for hypercholesterolemia,[43] ginkgo biloba for cognitive improvement in Alzheimer's disease,[44] and saw palmetto for improving urinary tract symptoms and flow rates.[45] There is far less evidence for the estimated 29,000 other dietary supplement products on the market, however.

## TRUTH IN LABELING

The FDA requires that specific information appear on a dietary supplement label. Labeling refers to the label as well as accompanying material that is used by a manufacturer to promote and market a specific product. It is important to understand that the types of claims that can be made on the labels of dietary supplements differ from those that can be made for prescription drugs. Whereas drug manufacturers may make the claim that their product will diagnose, cure, treat, mitigate, or prevent disease, such claims may not legally be made for dietary supplements. If a dietary supplement is marketed or promoted to cure, mitigate, or treat a disease, under current regulations the product would be considered to be an unauthorized new drug and the manufacturer would be in violation of the regulations and statutes regulating these products.

The label on a dietary supplement may include a health claim (describing a relationship between a food, food component, or dietary supplement ingredient and reducing the risk of a disease or health condition), a nutrient content claim (describing the relative amount of a nutrient or dietary substance in a product), or a structure/function claim (statement describing how a product may affect the organs or systems of the body, but it can not mention any specific disease).[46] Structure/function claims, for example, are broad claims that the product can support the structure or function of the body, such as glucosamine helps support healthy joints; St. John's wort is good for emotional well-being; and saw palmetto may alleviate the symptoms of benign prostatic hypertrophy. But, only drugs that have FDA-reviewed data on safety and efficacy may make disease-modifying claims. For example, it would be illegal to claim that St. John's wort treats mild to moderate depression because then the label would be mentioning a specific disease.

The product label is required to be truthful and not misleading. If the manufacturer says that its product addresses a nutrient deficiency, supports health, or reduces the risk of developing a health problem, then such claim must be followed in writing by the following: "This statement has not been evaluated by the Food and Drug Administration. This product is not intended to diagnose, treat, cure, or prevent any disease." Further, directions for use must be clearly stated. If the dietary ingredient is a botanical or herb, the scientific name of the plant or the plant part must be listed. If the product is a blend, the total weight of the blend and the components of the blend in order of predominance by weight must be listed. Nondietary ingredients (fillers, artificial colors, sweeteners, flavors) have to be listed by weight in descending order of predominance and by common name or proprietary blend. The word "supplement" must be included on the label, as must the net quantity of contents and the name and place of business of the manufacturer, packer, or distributor. The label of the supplement may contain a cautionary statement, but the manufacturer is not required to include one.[47]

Critics claim that dietary supplements overstate their importance and their impact on overall health, and evidence of many of the claimed benefits of certain dietary supplements have yet to meet a standard scientific criteria of credibility based on large-scale, double-blind, placebo-controlled trials. Indeed, numerous studies have documented scores of misleading claims made by the manufacturers about their products. A recent study of health claims made by herbal product manufacturers on the Internet found that 55% illegally claimed to treat, prevent, diagnose or cure specific diseases, despite regulations prohibiting such statements.[48] Examples include:

- Ginkgo Biloba's effects in improving circulation also contribute to its use for impotency and peripheral vascular insufficiency. Ginkgo treats depression, headaches, and memory loss ... and is also recommended for Alzheimer's disease, asthma, eczema and heart and kidney disorders.
- Valerian root is most effective in treating a wide range of stress conditions such as irritability, depression, fear, anxiety, nervous exhaustion, hysteria, delusions, and nervous tension ... and is useful for treating shingles, sciatica, neuralgia, multiple sclerosis, and epilepsy.

I am sure other examples can be found by searching the web by specific product.

Only two disease-related health claims have been approved by the FDA: folic acid reduces the risk of neural tube defects, and calcium supplementation reduces the risk of osteoporosis. What is somewhat alarming is the fact that more than half of those who search the Internet believe that "all" or "most" of the health information online is true.[49] This is especially troubling because studies have shown that a large percentage of Internet users search for health information and find credibility in what they read.[50] The volume of information on the Internet makes it difficult to monitor content. For the most part, much of the information found on the web pertaining to dietary supplement products is designed to promote the product without much regard to accuracy or truth in advertising. Although there are tools available for evaluating the quality of health-related Web sites, it is most unlikely that the consumer would regularly use such strategies while searching information on the Internet.

## QUALITY, SAFETY, AND STANDARDS ISSUES

It is difficult to determine the extent of side effects from dietary supplements because the surveillance systems are less extensive than those in place for pharmaceutical products. In contrast to the FDA approval process for pharmaceutical drugs, the FDA has to prove that a dietary supplement product is *not safe* in order to restrict its use or remove it from the market. Hampering the ability to get a better understanding of the extent of adverse events or side effects is the fact that dietary supplement manufacturers are not required by law to record, investigate, or forward information about adverse events associated with the use of their products to the FDA. Also, contributing to the underreporting of adverse effects of supplements is the fact that individuals taking these products may not report side effects to their physician (their physician may not even know that the patient is taking supplements). Although some adverse reactions to dietary supplements may manifest themselves fairly quickly, others such as kidney failure and other physiological reactions may be delayed and gradual in onset, making it difficult to relate the condition to the dietary supplement. Indeed, the relationship of the adverse event to the consumption of a supplement may not be readily apparent or even able to be proven. A review conducted by the Office of the Inspector General found that surveillance systems designed to detect adverse reactions to herbs, in particular, are inadequate and probably only detect less than 1% of all adverse events.[51]

Herbal products are often perceived as being safe because they are "natural." Yet, trying to ensure the safety of herbal products, in particular, is difficult because herbs contain potent bioactive substances. An important determinant of the safety of herbal supplements is the actual level of the toxic constituents in the herbal product. Studies have consistently shown that different brands of the same herb may vary considerably in their levels of characteristic constituents.[52] Different products prepared from the same herb may also show marked differences in biopharmaceutical quality.[53]

Herbal manufacturers are not required to submit evidence of safety to the FDA and the FDA does not "approve" or analyze herbal products before they are sold or marketed. The limited oversight in the United States is not shared in other countries. In Europe, for example, premarket approval is required for herbal medicinal products, and many European countries have established specific national regulations concerning the evaluation of herbal products.

Complicating the issue is that the processing of herbs (heating, boiling, etc.) may alter the pharmacological activity of the organic constituents. Time of harvest, soil conditions, and the part of the plant used individually and collectively can cause active ingredient levels to vary from batch to batch even with identical distillation procedures. Many serious and lethal adverse reactions have been reported among those who consumed herbal products, ephedra probably being the most publicized. Adverse reactions may occur through several different mechanisms, including direct toxic effects of the herb, allergic reactions to the product, and interactions with drugs or other supplements.[54]

Further, toxic contaminants including heavy metals, pesticides, and prescription drugs have been found in many supplement formulations. Commonly recommended mineral supplements such as calcium have been shown to include lead. Of twenty-three brands surveyed, eight had detectable levels of lead.[55] Calcium can prevent lead absorption thereby reducing the effect of contaminated calcium supplements on lead concentration in the blood.[56] A screening of 500 Chinese patent medicines showed that 10%–32% of the herbal products contained heavy metals or drugs not listed on the labels, and 10%–15% contained lead, mercury, or arsenic. Drug contaminants included ephedrine, recently banned by the FDA, and methyltestosterone (a male sex hormone that can cause liver cancer, congestive heart failure, and masculinization of female infants if a woman uses the product while pregnant).[57]

Compounding the safety and quality issues of dietary supplements is the lack of standardization among products. Whereas all drugs must comply with batch-to-batch standardization processes, dietary supplements are not required to be standardized. There is no legal or regulatory definition or procedure in the United States for standardization of dietary supplements despite the fact that the safe and effective use of any medicinal compound requires that each product sold has the same pharmacological and biological composition.[58] What seems to be the case is that active ingredients are often not known and certainly vary from manufacturer to manufacturer. Chemical analysis of supposedly standardized herbal preparations has revealed that many such products do not contain the amount of compound stated on the label, thus their potency may vary. One study found that ginsenoside levels (extracted from Panax ginseng) ranged from 30%–137% of the amount stated on the label.[59] Another study that analyzed fifty-nine preparations of Echinacea found that almost half did not contain the species listed on the label.[60] This wide variability makes it very difficult to evaluate the safety or efficacy of the products.

## FRAMEWORK FOR REGULATION OF THE INDUSTRY

Whereas quality control is quite stringent for drugs, the degree of quality control of a dietary supplement depends on the manufacturer or the supplier of the product, not the FDA. The manufacturer does not have to prove supplement quality per se, and the FDA is not required by law to analyze the content of dietary supplements. The FDA, however, is authorized to issue Good Manufacturing Practice (GMP) regulations for foods describing conditions under which dietary supplements must be prepared, packed, and stored. But, food GMPs do not always cover all issues of supplement quality. Some manufacturers voluntarily follow the FDA's GMPs for drugs, which are much stricter. But, in general, compared with the quality control for prescription drugs, quality control for dietary supplements is much less rigorous.

Part and parcel with quality is the need for oversight and regulation. The dietary supplement industry, however, has consistently and strongly resisted effective federal regulation, and has used its considerable political and economic clout to make sure its wishes were respected. Federal efforts to the contrary were consistently rebuffed. Legislation passed in the twentieth century largely ignored or exempted dietary supplements from effective oversight and regulation. The most striking example of the laissez-faire attitude towards the dietary supplement industry is best illustrated by the passage of the DSHEA of 1994, which is now the primary framework for the regulation of dietary supplements.

The DSHEA, which amended the Federal Food, Drug, and Cosmetic Act (FDCA) enacted in 1938, was intended to create a new regulatory framework for the safety and labeling of dietary supplements. The FDCA set the precedent for "after-the-fact" policy for foods, which implied that a food product was presumed safe unless the government proved that the food posed a reasonable possibility for injury in which case the government could remove the item from the market. Under the DSHEA, Congress opted against treating dietary supplements as drugs, rejecting the FDA's efforts to the contrary.

Congress' intent was to support two goals: (1) to facilitate consumer access to dietary supplements given that many consumers consume these products to help them maintain and improve their health, and (2) to give the FDA the authority to step in when safety problems arise and to ensure proper labeling of the product. Whether the intent and the actuality are the same is the subject of much debate.

Before the DSHEA was signed into law by President Clinton, dietary supplements were subject to the same regulatory requirements as other foods. When dietary supplements first were marketed, the FDA tried to regulate them using the procedures for new food ingredients, which was under this agency's purview. New food ingredients were presumed to be unsafe and had to be approved by the FDA before the product was made available to the consumer. The industry, however, did not want the FDA regulating their products and successfully blocked the FDA from assuming a strong regulatory role.

The DSHEA allowed dietary supplement manufacturers to market their products without receiving any premarket clearance from the FDA. Moreover, supplements sold in the United States before October 15, 1994, are not required to be reviewed by the FDA for safety because they are presumed to be safe based on their history of use. A manufacturer wishing to sell a supplement containing a new food ingredient (defined as one not marketed before October 15, 1994) needs only to notify the FDA 75 days before marketing and provide "some evidence" that the ingredient can "reasonably be expected to be safe." The FDA can refuse to allow the new ingredient to be marketed for safety reasons, but given the scant information provided about the product and the fact that so few adverse events are actually reported, the agency would be hard pressed to determine whether the product is indeed safe for human use or not.

When the FDA proposed that dietary supplements comply with food additive procedures, also under their purview, this proposal also was challenged by the industry. This premarket approval process would have been costly and time consuming to the dietary supplement industry. The matter was taken to court, and the FDA's position was unanimously rejected by the United States Court of Appeals for the Seventh Circuit and the United States Court of Appeals for the First Circuit.[61] The DSHEA explicitly exempts supplements from regulation as a food additive.

Basically, under the DSHEA, Congress adopted a similar regulatory stance for dietary supplements as that stipulated in the FDCA. Whereas food production companies must submit proof of safety for approval prior to marketing, FDA approval is not required for new supplement ingredients in the dietary supplement industry. A manufacturer, however, is responsible for determining that the dietary supplements it produces or distributes are safe and that any representations or claims made about them are substantiated by adequate evidence to show that they are not false or misleading. But, implicit in the act is that FDA approval for dietary supplements before they are marketed is *not* necessary. Further, a manufacturer does not have to provide the FDA with the evidence it relies on to substantiate safety or effectiveness before or after it markets its products. Manufacturers are not required to submit supporting data to the FDA in advance of marketing, as is required of prescription drug manufacturers, for example. Instead of manufacturers proving that their product is safe *before* they market and sell it, the FDA is responsible for proving that a supplement is unsafe *after* it has been on the market. The FDA is responsible for evaluating the evidence and tracking of adverse events after the fact.

Currently, there are no FDA regulations that are specific to dietary supplements that establish a minimum standard of practice for manufacturing dietary supplements. The manufacturer is responsible for establishing its own manufacturing practice guidelines to ensure that the dietary supplements it produces are safe and contain the ingredients listed on the label; but, as was stated earlier, this is not necessarily the case. The DSHEA's deregulatory approach essentially ignores the risks that these products could pose to consumers. In reality, the DSHEA freed the industry from effective oversight by the FDA. The DSHEA's highly deregulatory approach won effusive praise from the industry, which professed strong belief in the ability of consumers to make intelligent choices about supplement use. Critics were dubious that the typical consumer could exercise informed decision making regarding the safety and effectiveness of the products. Given that the labels on many products are misleading or inaccurate, even assuming that the consumer could make an intelligent decision, the consumer is not given all the information needed to make a determination whether the product is "good" for them or not.

The act restricted the FDA's control over dietary supplements and made it easier for manufacturers to make health claims and harder for regulatory agencies to prevent them from so doing. Manufacturers are bound by the Federal Trade Commission (FTC), which regulates advertising, including infomercials, for dietary supplements and most other products sold to the consumer. How effective the FTC is as a watchdog is debatable. Its "Operation Cure All," which was intended to educate consumers about recognizing health fraud, was targeted at Internet supplement vendors who made illegal health claims. A study evaluating this program found that 55% of retail Web sites accessed through the most common search engines still claimed that supplements could treat or prevent specific diseases (clearly against the law), and 52% of Web sites omitted the standard federal disclaimer (also against the law).[62]

Many private organizations have tried to fill the gap in consumer education and quality assurance since the DSHEA was passed. Most compile research on safety and efficacy for patient and physician education. The Dietary Supplement Verification Program (DSVP), for example, accepts *voluntary* submission of products by manufacturers and awards a U.S. Pharmacopeia National Formulary certification if the product contains the ingredients stated on the label, has the declared amount of ingredients, has been screened for harmful contaminants, and has been manufactured by safe sanitary and well-controlled procedures.[63] Although being awarded this certificate means that a product is manufactured consistently from batch to batch and is not contaminated, it does not ensure that the product is safe or useful.

In summary, the DSHEA essentially gave the dietary supplement industry carte blanche in its production/manufacture and marketing of its products. Basically, manufacturers can make certain claims without proof of safety and efficacy. To a large extent, dietary supplements are subject to lower safety standards than are food additives, and consumers are provided with more information about the composition and nutritional value of food sold in supermarkets than they are about the ingredients and potential hazards of botanical medicines, which are unregulated and can pose serious health hazards.

## NOW WHAT?

A significant number of new dietary supplement products have appeared in the marketplace since the U.S. Congress passed the DSHEA. At the time DSHEA was enacted, an estimated 600 U.S. dietary supplement manufacturers marketed about 4,000 products. A decade later, more than 29,000 different dietary supplements are now available to consumers. Some, of course, have genuine therapeutic potential, but others have not lived up to the hype or claims made by the manufacturer. Numerous dietary supplements have been shown not to be therapeutically beneficial or effective. But, since manufacturers are not legally required to provide specific information about safety and effectiveness before marketing their products, and since adverse events associated with dietary supplements are recorded only through voluntary reporting (an inherently weak form of surveillance to be sure), the ability of the FDA to effectively monitor risks and adverse events is severely limited.

The limited oversight in the United States is in stark contrast to that in other countries. In most European countries, for example, premarket approval is required for herbal products and there are established specific national registries regarding the evaluation of these products. The European Union also issued multiple directives on manufacturing and quality testing of herbal products. Japan and China regulate these products as pharmaceuticals.[64]

In the United States, some have called for the repeal of the DSHEA.[65] Since this is not likely to happen in the near term, what steps should be taken to ensure that the products produced and marketed are safe? Safety research needs to become a priority in this industry to clarify potential hazards and risks of the products. That dietary supplements are derived from natural substances does not render them invariably safe. Unsafe products remain on market shelves because consumers and regulators are not hearing about adverse events. Increasing consumer confidence in the products is best served by focusing on product safety rather than on misleading claims. There needs to be better labeling of these products. Each product's label should identify the substances in the product as well as the concentration of such substances. There also needs to be better standardization of the batches produced.

Many have called for a comprehensive register of dietary supplements, as well as a strengthened surveillance system that would mandate reporting of adverse events.[66] Others have called for mandatory registration of supplement manufacturers and vendors, required evidence of efficacy and safety before marketing, and standardization of purity and potency.[67] Basically, what is needed is that the burden of proof be placed on the manufacturer. Just as the manufacturers benefit from sales of their products, they should also bear the burden of conducting rigorous safety testing, as is required in the pharmaceutical industry.

# 9

# Silicone Breast Implants: Misconceptions, Misinterpretations, and Mistakes

In 1977, Mariann Hopkins underwent a bilateral mastectomy as a result of fibrocystic disease of the breasts, a relatively benign condition in which one or more cysts form in the breast. Immediately following the mastectomies, Ms. Hopkins underwent reconstruction with Dow Corning silicone gel-filled implants. From February 1978 through March 1979, she was evaluated for a variety of symptoms and her physicians told her that she might be suffering from mixed connective tissue disease. The symptoms of this debilitating and lifelong disease eventually forced her to quit her job in 1986. That same year, she had to replace her implants because one of them had ruptured.

Ms. Hopkins sued Dow Corning.[1] At trial, she alleged defective design, defective manufacturing, breach of express and implied warranty, fraud, and failure to warn her that silicone gel breast implants may cause connective tissue diseases. Three expert witnesses who testified on her behalf analyzed the Dow Corning laboratory studies and introduced anecdotal information into the court proceeding. The defense also had experts who opined that Ms. Hopkins' symptoms began prior to her receiving the implants. Based on the "evidence" presented, the jury ruled on behalf of the plaintiff and awarded Ms. Hopkins $7.34 million. Dow Corning immediately appealed the verdict arguing that the plaintiff's evidence was not admissible. The appeals court not only reaffirmed the verdict, but also issued a harsh statement concerning Dow Corning's conduct in exposing thousands of women to a substance that may cause painful and debilitating diseases.

A closer look at this case, however, raises doubts whether the court reached a proper conclusion. The testimony presented by the plaintiff expert witnesses was questioned for validity, and their credentials were questioned as well. Neither was an epidemiologist or an expert in biostatistics. In the absence of an understood biological mechanism or specific medical test or tests, an epidemiologist or biostatistician would be the likely experts who could give scientifically accurate testimony about the possibility of Ms. Hopkins' autoimmune disorder being causally related to her silicone gel breast implants. In light of the absence of good epidemiological evidence, why, then, did the jury decide in favor of the plaintiff?

## THE SILICONE BREAST IMPLANT SAGA

Silicone gel breast implants were taken off the market in the United States fifteen years after Ms. Hopkins' surgery. During this time, numerous studies were conducted to determine the safety of silicone breast implants. Well over one million women had had silicone implant surgery, and over the decades there were reports that linked implant ruptures to autoimmune problems in some individuals. Numerous lawsuits were filed against the manufacturers. Yet, the story behind these actions masks what turned out to be an interesting tale of judicial misuse of evidence that led not only to the financial ruin of one of the manufacturers of the product, but also to untold emotional distress for many women.

Essentially, the silicone breast implant saga illustrates how the American legal system failed to meet the challenge of separating scientific facts from anecdotal testimony, and how difficult it was for juries to differentiate scientifically valid evidence from "junk" science and emotionally laden personal stories. The lessons to be learned from this emotionally charged issue are many, but the one that supersedes the others is that the scientific approach to assessing risk and causality must take precedent in the courtroom. "Junk science" has no place in the legal system. This chapter focuses on the silicone gel breast implant controversy and tries to piece together the complex scientific and legal issues that are so central to the case. In order to understand the complex issues of the case, it is imperative to have an understanding of the epidemiological concept of cause and effect.

## CAUSE AND EFFECT ISSUES

The means and methods of determining scientific truth differ from judicial methods. In science, data-based tests and studies are conducted; no one test or finding can be considered to be the final word, as findings must be validated by other studies. Lawsuits involving complex health issues rely on scientific evidence and expert witness testimony, but determining that both the evidence presented and the expert testimony are valid and relevant has been a source of controversy and contention. Part of the problem has been juxtaposing legal requirements with the epidemiological/scientific evidence.

In order to fully appreciate the events that led to the removal of silicone gel breast implants from the market, it is important to have a general understanding of epidemiological methods. Epidemiological findings are often introduced into court cases, especially in product liability cases, but causality in epidemiology is not always interpreted the same in the law. In the court system, the adversarial process often determines truth: plaintiff versus defense. In cases involving product liability, for example, the defendant (the manufacturer) must argue that its product did not harm the plaintiff. Two types of causation must be established: general and specific.

Epidemiology focuses on the question of general causation (Is the agent capable of causing disease?) rather than that of specific causation (Did the agent cause the disease in the individual?). Indeed, epidemiological studies cannot offer specific causation and cannot provide direct evidence that a particular plaintiff was injured by exposure to a particular substance.[2] Yet, the plaintiff must establish that not only is the defendant's agent capable of causing disease, but that it did cause the disease. Epidemiology's usefulness to individual plaintiffs relates more directly to issues of elevated risk rather than actual occurrence.

When an epidemiologist evaluates whether a cause–effect relationship exists between an agent and a disease, the term causation is used in a way similar to, but not identical with, the *sine qua non test* used in the law for cause in fact ("but for"). An increase in disease would not have occurred in the group ("but for") had the individuals not been exposed to the agent, for example. While perhaps logical in the law, the practice of drawing inferences about causation in epidemiology can be complicated and controversial. One part of the issue is that epidemiology relies on population-based data and does not draw conclusions specific to one individual. Epidemiology as a science is rarely able to provide experimental proof as can be done in the laboratory. Rather, the epidemiological process relies on causal inference; that is, accumulating evidence of a relationship between health or disease and other factors and then statistically assessing the strength of the association between the exposure and the disease. Association refers to the degree of statistical dependence between two or more events or variables. Events are said to be associated when they occur more frequently together than one would expect by chance. Epidemiological studies help assess the strength or absence of an association between an agent and a disease, but even the most carefully designed studies do not demonstrate more than a high probability of a causal relationship. It is very rare to be 100% certain that exposure A caused disease B.

Causation, as defined in epidemiology, denotes an event, condition, characteristic, or agent that is a necessary element of a set of other events that produce an outcome such as a disease. That is, one gets malaria by being bitten by an infected mosquito. Being bitten is a necessary link in the causal chain that results in an outcome (malaria). Causation, however, remains a matter of judgment based on available evidence. Concluding that factor A is causally associated with disease B must be based on a firm statistical interpretation of the data. Potential sources of bias and confounding such as inappropriate sample selection or error in measuring exposure among those included in the study must be identified and assessed. There is a danger that bias and confounding may exaggerate, dilute, or mask a true association.

Epidemiological evidence focuses on identifying an agent or agents (a drug, medical device, a microorganism, and substance) that is/are associated with an increased risk of disease in groups of individuals. Epidemiological studies focus on identifying those individuals who might be at higher risk of disease after being exposed to an agent and statistically quantify this risk. There are guidelines and criteria that help epidemiologists make a judgment about causation. For example, the stronger the association between an agent and a disease, the more likely it is that the relationship is causal and less likely that it is due to bias or confounding. But, other issues must be satisfied to avoid making a mistake in assumption of causality. Is there a logical temporal sequence between agent and disease (did the malaria develop *after* the mosquito bite)? Do the findings make biological sense? Is there a logical dose-response relationship between agent and disease? Have other studies found similar findings? Have alternative explanations been ruled out?

## ASSESSING RISK AND ASSESSING BURDEN OF PROOF

The strength of an association between exposure and disease is statistically calculated. The relative risk and the odds ratio, for example, are measures of association that give an indication of the degree to which the risk of a disease increases when individuals are exposed to a specific agent. A score of 1 implies no association (risk in the exposed population is the same as the risk in the unexposed population). Anything higher than 1 implies elevated risk; for example, a relative risk of 3.0 indicates that the risk of disease in the exposed group is three times higher than the risk of disease in the unexposed group. A relative risk of 1.5 would mean a 50% increase in likelihood, but it would also mean that for a given individual who developed the disease, there would be a two-thirds probability that the illness was not caused by the exposure. Anything less than 1 implies a protective or curative effect.

In tort law, the plaintiff must convince the jury that the defendant is guilty by a "preponderance of evidence" and that the plaintiff's lawyer must establish that not only is the defendant's agent capable of causing disease, but that it did cause the disease and that this fact is more likely than not true. But, the concept can be tricky to apply to medico-legal matters. In the past, there often was a dichotomy between what the plaintiff's lawyer would like to say and what the epidemiological data would allow the lawyer to say. What then is acceptable legal proof of causation based on epidemiological evidence?

The standard in civil court is "more probably than not." Only conclusions from a study finding a relative risk greater than 2 can be used to argue that it is more probably than not that the exposure caused illness. The courts have required a 50% plus standard to answer the question of burden of proof. That is, the threshold for concluding that an agent is more likely than not to be the cause of a disease is a relative risk or an odds ratio of 2 or more. This would imply a greater than 50% likelihood that an exposed individual's disease was caused by the agent. The jury does not need to be certain that the agent or exposure caused the disease, only that they are more than 50% confident in their conclusion. But, other factors may play an important legal role in determining the specifics of causation. There may be factors peculiar to the plaintiff such as a family history of the disease, which may make it more difficult to support the inference that an agent is more likely than not responsible for the plaintiff's disease.

## SCIENTIFIC VALIDITY IN THE COURTROOM

The courts have found that determining causation in tort cases is far more difficult than in cases involving assaults or automobile accidents. Because plaintiffs are required to prove causation in order to recover monetary awards, expert testimony is usually needed in tort cases. A plaintiff in a tort case is obligated to prove that his or her claims are more likely true than not. Because of the unique nature of many tort claims, this can be a difficult task, even if the plaintiff is suffering from a serious illness.

A plaintiff's attempt to prove a direct cause-and-effect relationship may be complicated by the difficulty in identifying the substance that caused the plaintiff's injury. For example, when chemical and manufacturing plants dispose of hazardous waste, they generally dispose of many different substances simultaneously over a long period of time. These substances then intermingle and may migrate together in water or evaporate together into the air. Therefore, although a plaintiff may be able to demonstrate that he or she was exposed to this group of toxic substances, the intermingling effect of the substances can make it virtually impossible for the plaintiff to identify a particular substance as having caused the plaintiff's injury. Assuming that a plaintiff can identify the agent or exposure, a plaintiff still may have difficulty proving that that agent or exposure caused his or her injury. The source or cause of many diseases can be very difficult to prove conclusively. There may be other causal factors that may make it virtually impossible for a plaintiff to prove that the defendant's product or negligent activity caused the plaintiff's disease.[3]

Another difficult problem is determining whether expert testimony is based on scientifically valid principles. In the past, judicial approaches toward the use of epidemiological evidence often were inconsistent, or worse, incorrect largely as a result of an inability to accept or recognize epidemiology's limitations in assessing causation. In order to ensure that the evidence proffered is not based on personal opinions, over the years, the courts have tried to set standards upon which testimony must be assessed.

In 1923, in *Frye v. United States*, the Court of Appeals of the District of Columbia established that the scientific principle must be "generally accepted" in its field to become the basis for expert testimony.[4] Even thought no explanation was offered by the court as to how to apply the standard, this ruling set the conduct of science in the courtroom for the next fifty years![5] The Frye test was not immune to criticism; principles that are hard to test and take many years to produce results may not be deemed "generally acceptable." It was up to the court to determine whether the technique and principles employed had received general acceptance in the scientific community. Basically, the Frye test tried to provide a framework in which to exclude "junk science" or patently false testimony opined by "experts."

In 1975, the Federal Rules of Evidence were enacted, and these rules for federal courts relaxed the standards under which scientific evidence could be heard. These rules did away with the "general acceptance" concept and placed the judge in the responsible position of determining which evidence is valid, reliable, and relevant. By doing so, judges were placed in a position of authority to sift through evidence before being presented in court. In reality, however, some courtrooms allowed virtually all of the evidence to be presented to the jury, thus putting jurors in a position of deciding the validity and relevancy of the testimony.

In the silicone gel breast implant cases, for example, plaintiffs asked the Supreme Court to decide whether the Federal Rules of Evidence had superseded the general acceptance standards of Frye, arguing under Rule 702 that it is up to the judge to decide whether the witness will present scientific knowledge, whether this knowledge will assist the jury, and whether the witnesses are qualified as experts. Rule 702 requires that two preliminary determinations be made by the trial court. First, the proffered witness must be qualified as an expert by knowledge, skill, experience, training, or education. Second, the proffered expert's opinion, inference, or other testimony must be based on scientific, technical, or other specialized knowledge that will assist the "trier of fact" to understand the evidence or determine a fact in issue. The Supreme Court ruled that the Federal Rules do supersede the Frye standard and that the judge does have a duty to screen the evidence.

In 1993, the case of *Daubert v. Merrell Dow Pharmaceuticals* was brought before the Supreme Court on appeal.[6] The *Daubert* case involved claims by a mother of two children born with physical defects that the prescription drug Bendectin, given to prevent nausea, caused the birth defects. Over 17.5 million women had taken Bendectin as an antinausea medication for morning sickness. Scores of studies failed to show an association between Bendectin and birth defects, yet Merrell Dow spent in excess of $100 million defending itself against lawsuits alleging that the drug had been responsible for fetal abnormalities. Experts for Daubert said that Merrell Dow's animal studies provided evidence that the drug caused birth defects. Merrell Dow's experts interpreted the findings differently.

In 1993, the Supreme Court directed a lower court to determine whether the scientific testimony was admissible under the Federal Rules of Evidence. The Ninth Circuit Court ruled that the plaintiffs had not produced acceptable evidence that had achieved general acceptance in the scientific community. That is, the plaintiff's epidemiological analyses of the studies were ruled inadmissible because the results had not been published or been subject to peer review.

The Supreme Court analyzed the principles, rules of evidence, and procedures governing expert testimony based on scientific knowledge. The court determined that the judges were responsible for ensuring that evidence be admitted only if it is both relevant and reliable. The *Daubert* decision, as it is commonly known, held that judges have a duty to screen evidence. The Supreme Court decision also emphasized that a trial court must determine at the outset whether the reasoning or methodology underlying the testimony is scientifically valid. This opinion emphasized the jury's role and the trial judge's responsibility to keep unreliable evidence ("junk science") out of the courtroom.

The Daubert case was concerned with scientific evidence and scientific credibility for research to be admissible under Federal Rules of Evidence. Whereas under the *Frye* ruling, the general acceptance standard meant that the scientific community played a major role in what would be admitted into a court of law, the Daubert decision entrusted the judges with that role. Judges would be the gatekeepers who would ensure that the scientific testimony or evidence was not only relevant but also reliable.

The Daubert standard has become the gold standard for evaluating scientific evidence and for determining what evidence would be admissible in court. This landmark case has done much to screen unproved scientific evidence, ill-founded or speculative theories, and anecdotal opinions that are not verifiable from the courtroom.

The Bendectin case has many parallels with the silicone litigation.[7] As in the *Daubert v. Merrell Dow* case, the silicone gel breast implant litigation illustrates how science and the law can, at times, work at cross-purposes.

## BREAST IMPLANTS: A LITTLE BIT OF HISTORY

Until the mid-twentieth century, a variety of substances were used to enhance the size of the breast including glass balls, ground rubber, ox cartilage, sponges made from polyvinyl alcohol and plyether, as well as many natural substances. Understandably, adverse reactions to the introduction of these sorts of products into the body were common.

Early attempts to use silicone in breast implants date from the 1940s. Silicone is a synthetic polymer consisting of silicon, oxygen, and carbon side chains. It may be in the form of a solid, a liquid, or a gel, depending on the nature of chemical cross-links. The use of liquid silicone injection for breast augmentation, for example, was in vogue until complications, including infection, inflammation, scarring, and breast disfigurement, helped put a stop to this practice in the early 1970s. Other medical uses of silicone include components of cardiac pacemakers, intraocular lenses, syringes, ventricular shunts, antacids, and artificial joints.[8]

Breast implants, both silicone and saline, have been an integral part of breast surgery for decades. They have been used after a mastectomy, to correct breast and chest deformities, and for augmentation. The primary difference between silicone and saline implants is that the latter are filled with a sterile saltwater solution and the former with a gel. Whereas the gel-filled implants are prefilled by the manufacturer, the saline implants are filled via a valve after being placed in the body. Silicone gel generally was preferred because gel gave the breast a more natural feel. Also, a saline implant is less likely to produce as aesthetic a result when there is little existing breast tissue to cover it.

The first breast augmentation using silicone gel-filled implants dates from the early 1960s. Plastic surgeons Thomas Cronin and Frank Gerow, working with Dow Corning, conceived the idea of a thin silicone elastomer shell that would be filled with a liquid or gel material. The barrier coating of breast implant shells of special silicone elastomer was designed to minimize the migration of gel from the implants.

Smooth thick shells and firm gel characterized the first generation of breast implants often with a Dacron patch on the back to help them adhere to the chest wall. These devices had low rupture rates, but often caused contractures (scar tissue contracts and this effect serves to squeeze the implant into a hard, round ball resulting in visible bulges in the upper part of the breast) and had a high gel bleed rate (implant shell remains intact but there is a diffusion of small molecules of liquid components of silicone gel through the intact shell of the implant into the body).

The second generation of breast implants dates from the mid-1970s through the 1980s. The designers of the implants strove to create implants that would mimic the feel of natural breasts as much as possible. To achieve this feel, the shells of the implants were smooth and thin and the gel was softer and more liquid than the earlier designs. However, there was little attention paid to the safety of the product, and the newer generation of implants was associated with all of the same problems as those of the first generation. The rupture and deflation rates were actually higher than the earlier versions.

In the third generation, dating from the 1980s to the mid-1990s, the focus shifted to lowering the complications rate. The shells were made stronger to resist rupture and were also coated on the inside in an effort to reduce the gel bleed rate. The shells were textured, which helped to reduce the incidence of contracture. By the end of the 1990s, approximately 1.5 to 1.8 million women in the United States had had implant surgery. Of this, 70% of these implants were performed for augmentation and 30% for reconstruction.[9]

Breast implants are not lifetime devices; they are not expected to last forever. Moreover, placement of any foreign substance, product, or device in the body carries risks. Silicone is a relatively bland substance and is considered to be one of the least reactive and fairly nontoxic biomaterials. Although tests showed little reaction to the compound, there always is the possible risk of local inflammatory and scarring reactions as well as infection. The longer the implants are in place, the higher the risk of complications. While most women with silicone breast implants initially did not experience adverse effects, there were some who developed serious health problems.

## HEALTH RISKS

The first nonscientific reports identifying cases of connective tissue disorders (systemic lupus erythematosus, rheumatoid arthritis, scleroderma or systemic sclerosis, polymyalgia, fibromyalgia, and atypical connective tissue disease, among others) were noted in Japan in the 1960s. These reports primarily identified Japanese women who had received injections of paraffin or adulterated silicone, but not gel-filled prostheses. Although these reports were considered not to be relevant to American women, considerable research was conducted to assess health risks associated with the silicone gel-filled breast implant. Early animal and cell-based studies on the toxicity of silicone concluded that there did not seem to be long-term systemic toxic effects from silicone gel implants or from unsuspected compounds in these gels detected by these experiments.[10] In the mid- to late-1980s, an animal study showed that silicone gel implants could cause cancer in rats, but it was concluded that the cancers seen were caused by a well-described mechanism that was only relevant to these test animals.[11]

An Australian study published in 1982 first raised the question of a connection between connective tissue disease and silicone gel breast implant patients.[12] Subsequently, other studies were conducted to investigate this link. After a study investigating the link between silicone gel breast implants and disease was published in the *Journal of the American Medical Association*,[13] the American medical community began to consider the possibility that silicone exposure might cause disease in some patients. Prior to this publication, there were only a dozen isolated case reports in the medical literature. Case reports are not analytic studies; they do not test hypotheses; they cannot show elevated risk. But, case reports can raise questions about an experience of a small group of individuals who present with similar symptoms or a similar diagnosis. Because the symptoms reported were expected to occur in some percentage of women anyway, and because the number of cases was so low, the link between symptoms and silicone implants was thought to be coincidental and not causal. Nevertheless, the medical community saw the existence of these reports as a reason to investigate further. The report also raised several issues about the deficiencies and missed opportunities on the part of the Food and Drug Administration (FDA). The report characterized the FDA as placing an excessive emphasis on anecdotal opinion rather than on scientifically proved data.

## EVIDENCE OF SAFETY OF SILICONE GEL BREAST IMPLANTS

There have been many international panels and committees formed to look at the safety of silicone gel breast implants. In the United States, the Institute of Medicine (IOM) assembled a committee to review peer-reviewed, published scientific literature dating from the early 1990s (see reference 9). The IOM committee was composed of experts in many fields, and care was taken to avoid conflicts of interest because of the highly political and controversial nature of the issue. In the United Kingdom, the Independent Review Group (IRG) was formed to review evidence relating to the possible health risks associated with the silicone gel breast implants.[14] Groups and committees were set up in Canada[15] and in France[16] to study the issue. While the conclusions of these reports were consistent with those reached by the British and Americans, the Canadian report commented that while a number of biological problems have been reported (capsule development, capsular contracture, silicone infiltration of lymph nodes), neither the frequency nor the health impact of these were known, and their relationship to possible associated disease states was undefined. Associations with autoimmune diseases were based solely on case reports.

The following summarizes the key findings from these scientific blue ribbon panels, as well as from reports issued by the manufacturers. It is not intended to be a comprehensive account, rather the intention is to present a concise summary of the epidemiological findings. For a more in-depth report, please refer to the IOM and the IRG reports, as well as Angell's book, *Science on Trial: The Clash of Medical Evidence and the Law in the Breast Implant Case*.[17]

### Connective Tissue Disorders

Litigants argued that silicone can stimulate the immune system and that the silicone implants caused a variety of immunologically mediated diseases, including autoimmune disease and connective tissue disease. The defense experts countered that the clinical criteria for atypical connective tissue disease are vague, subjective, and inclusive of "symptoms" that are equally common in healthy individuals. While not denying that some women did indeed suffer adverse effects from their silicone implants, the epidemiological studies evaluating women with breast implants showed no increased risk of defined connective tissue diseases among the implant recipients compared with a similar group of women from the same area who did not have implants. Women who developed complications, the most common being systemic sclerosis (scleroderma), also alleged that their implants were the cause of their complications. Epidemiological research, however, found no statistically significant increase in scleroderma. That is, there was no evidence that the incidence of scleroderma in women with breast implants was any higher than in the general population (see Table 9.1). This is not to imply that some women with breast implants have not experienced connective tissue and related disorders. It only

**Table 9.1**
**The risk of connective tissue disease associated with silicone breast implants**

| Reference | Relative Risk/Odds Ratio |
| --- | --- |
| Burns et al., *J Rheumatology* 23:1904–1911. 1996 | 0.95 (95% confidence interval [CI]: 0.21–4.36) |
| Edworthy et al., *J Rheumatology* 25:254–60. 1998 | 1.0 (95% CI: 0.45–2.22) |
| Englert et al., *Australian NZ J Med* 26:349–55. 1996 | 1.0 (95% CI: 0.16–6.16) |
| Friis et al., *Annals Plastic Surgery* 39:1–8. 1997 | Cosmetic: 1.1 (95% CI: 0.2–3.4) |
|  | Reconstructive: 1.3 (95% CI: 0.5–3.6) |
| Gabriel et al., *New Engl J Med* 330:1697–1702. 1994 | 1.1 (95% CI: 0.37–3.23) |
| Giltay et al., *Annals Rheum Dis* 53:194–196. 1994 | 0.44 (no CI) |
| Goldman et al., *J Clin Epi* 48:571–582. 1995 | 0.52 (95% CI: 0.27–0.92) |
| Hennekens et al., *JAMA* 275 (8): 616–621. 1996 | 1.24 (95% CI: 1.08–1.41) |
| Hochberg et al., *Arthritis and Rheum* 39:1125–31. 1996 | 1.07 (95% CI: 0.53–2.13) |
| Park et al., *Plastic Reconstr Surg* 101:261–267. 1998 | 0.42 (95% CI: 0.1–15.63) |
| Sanchez-Guerrero et al., *New Engl J Med* 332:1666–1670. 1995 | 0.6 (95% CI: 0.2–2.01) |
| Schusterman et al., *Annals Plastic Surg* 31:1–6. 1993 | 1.08 (95% CI: 0.1–17.2) |
| Strom et al., *J Clin Epi* 47:1211–1214. 1994 | 4.5 (95% CI: 0.2–27.3) |
| Williams et al., *Arthritis and Rheum* 40:437–440. 1997 | 0.74 (80% CI: 0.2–2.02) |

means that there is not a statistically elevated risk of developing these disorders that can be attributed to silicone gel breast implants.

Most of the cases reported in the literature are suggestive of connective tissue diseases, but the symptoms and laboratory values are not precise enough to diagnose these women with the diseases. There also is no conclusive evidence that silicone gel breast implants caused these symptoms. Many of the women experienced rashes, fatigue, dry eyes, or chronic flu-like symptoms, which, while associated with connective tissue diseases, also could be brought on by depression, allergies, and stress. Further, these symptoms may be present in individuals without connective tissue disease or without breast implants.

One of the largest studies to investigate the issue was conducted by Hennekens et al. (400,000 women; 11,000 with breast implants), and findings showed that over a ten-year period, women with breast implants were 1.24 times more likely to report having a connective tissue disorder compared with women without breast implants, a very weak association at best. In an effort to address misclassification issues resulting from self-reported conditions, a medical records validation of the conditions led to a recalculation of risk estimate of 1.19, which is not statistically significant. The vast majority of women with implants will *not* develop defined autoimmune-related disorders as a result of having an implant.[18] Further, a meta-analysis of studies published in the 1990s found no evidence of an association between breast implants in general, or silicone gel breast implants specifically. The conclusion was that breast implants appear to have a minimal effect on the number of women in whom connective tissue diseases develop.[19]

Further, the IOM's review of seventeen epidemiological reports of connective tissue disease in women with silicone breast implants conclusively found no elevated risk.[20] The IRG came to the same conclusion based on their review of the literature.[21] Some scientists believed that it was possible for the immune system to create antibodies that were specific to silicone itself, or to silicone modified human proteins. To that end, researchers tried to develop tests that looked for antibodies against silicone that may be present in the blood of silicone gel breast implant cases. The IOM committee reviewed many such tests and concluded that none was capable of detecting antibodies against silicone. In fact, there were positive results with any blood test, regardless of whether an individual had been exposed to silicone or not.

In summary, the epidemiological evidence showed none or only a weak association between connective tissue diseases and silicone gel breast implants.

## Breast Cancer

Perhaps more frightening to women was the suggestion that breast implants could cause breast cancer. Early animal experiments, where implants were placed in rodents to evaluate safety, showed development of solid-state tumors (sarcomas). These tumors, however, are quite different from the tumors commonly found in human breasts. Further, it had been shown that rodents develop sarcomas in response to a great variety of solid substances, not just silicone. Hence, this suggests that silicone is not specifically cancer-inducing in mice.[22]

There were, however, numerous case reports and anecdotes suggesting that women who had been injected with silicone for breast augmentation developed breast cancer.

As discussed earlier, these reports cannot be considered scientifically valid and should not form the basis for a lawsuit. Numerous studies that had looked at the carcinogenicity of silicone gel breast implants uniformly concluded that there was no association between breast implants and breast cancer. The IOM committee conducted an exhaustive review of reports and studies that specifically looked at the association of cancer, including sarcomas and carcinomas,

**Table 9.2**
**Selected studies of silicone breast implants and cancer**

| Reference | Standardized incidence ratio or odds ratio (adjusted) |
| --- | --- |
| Brinton et al., *Am J Epi* 141:S85. 1995 | No association found |
| Bryant et al., *New Engl J Med* 332:1535–9. 1995 | 0.76 (95% CI: 0.6–1.0) |
| Deapen et al., *Plastic Reconstr Surg* 99:1346. 1997 | 0.63 (95% CI: 0.4–0.9) |
| Friis et al., *Internatl J Cancer* 71:956–958. 1997 | 1.0 (95% CI: 0.4–2.0) |
| McLaughlin et al., *J Natl Cancer Inst* 90:156. 1998 | 0.7 (95% CI: 0.4–1.1) |

with breast implants and concluded that there was no evidence to suggest that women with breast implants had a higher incidence of cancer than those women without implants (see Table 9.2). In fact, some of the long-term cohort studies, some following women for two decades or more after their implant surgery, found fewer breast cancers than expected.[23]

### Polyurethane Implants and Cancer Risk

Gel-filled implants have a layer of polyurethane foam coating the silicone envelope. An estimated 10% of implants are of this type. However, the manufacturer voluntarily removed these implants from the market after questions were raised about a possible cancer risk from the chemical breakdown of the polyurethane foam, whose purpose was to reduce the chance of capsular contraction. One of the breakdown products, 2-toluene diamine (TDA), is considered a probable animal carcinogen and a possible human one. Studies, however, showed that TDA does not end up in the systems of women with polyurethane implants.[24]

### Neurological Disease

There had been suggestions that silicone gel-filled breast implants could be the cause of a variety of neurological effects of a multiple sclerosis type syndrome. Animal studies, however, did not support the anecdotal reports that silicone is a cause of neurological disease. The Practice Committee of the American Academy of Neurology, in 1997, reviewed the available literature and concluded that there was no support for the hypothesis. That is, there is no association or causal relationship between silicone gel-filled breast implants and neurological disorders.[25]

### Allergic Reaction

Silicone, which has been used in the manufacture of numerous medical devices and products for decades, does not appear to be associated with the development of allergies. One could develop antibodies to the silicone, but the presence of these antibodies does not indicate disease.[26]

### Risk of Breast Feeding

Breast implants made of silicone materials generate two issues of concern relative to breastfeeding: (1) do the implants leak silicone compounds into human milk? and (2) do the implants cause some type of immunologic disease in the infant?[27] That is, do women with silicone gel-filled implants who breast-feed pass autoimmune problems to their children? A Dow Corning study found silicone in breast milk, but it also found essentially the same amount of silicone in breast milk regardless of whether the mother had implants or not.[28] Researchers concluded that there did not appear to be any evidence to support the view that women with implants should avoid breastfeeding.

### Summary of the Epidemiological Evidence

Case-control and cohort studies published from 1970 to 1998 generally found that the level of increased risk for all disorders was small, and few could provide support for any increased risk of connective tissue disease. In light of the epidemiological and toxicological evidence, it appears that diseases and conditions such as autoimmune disorders are no more common in women with breast implants than in women without breast implants. In fact, given that millions of women have had implants, by chance alone it would be expected that a proportion would develop connective tissue diseases, cancer, neurological diseases, and possibly other systemic complaints or conditions.

Yet, approximately 400,000 women have joined class action lawsuits against silicone implant manufacturers. An additional 20,000 to 30,000 others chose to litigate individually. Assuming an average award of $2 million on the basis of verdicts for either the plaintiff or defense, $40 to $60 billion was at stake in this litigation, independent of legal fees.[29] Given the accumulation of evidence showing no elevation in risk, how did the courts initially arrive at decision in favor of the plaintiffs? What changed the tide in favor of the defense?

### BURDEN OF PROOF IN THE SILICONE GEL BREAST IMPLANT LITIGATION

In order to render a "proper" legal decision, the court must somehow make sure that the evidence presented is scientifically accurate, accepted, and understood by the judge and jury. Without proper scientific evidence, finding a party guilty or liable would violate the spirit of the law and undermine the purpose of the courts. In many of the early silicone gel breast implant cases, Daubert or Frye standards were not applied or applied inconsistently. For example, in *Hall v. Baxter Health Care Corp*, the judge did not rule on the admissibility of studies relied on by the plaintiffs' experts, rather he ruled on the experts' opinions themselves. Upon review, the testimony of these experts was excluded as it was deemed that the plaintiffs simply failed to meet a well-established legal standard.[30]

From 1991 to 1995, both plaintiffs and the defense won as many cases as they lost. From 1996 on, however, there was a noticeable shift in verdicts in favor of the defense. By this time, more epidemiological studies were published, and based on the new evidence upon which Daubert standards were enforced, the defense tended to win the cases primarily because the scientific studies consistently and convincingly showed weak associations or no associations between the gel-filled implants and disease (see Table 9.3). The Daubert standards were enforced, thus screening out inappropriate evidence and testimony.

How have subsequent court decisions been affected post 1996? Whereas state courts had differed in their interpretations of *Daubert*, especially interpreting appropriate standards of review for the judge's decisions regarding the admissibility of scientific evidence, the Supreme Court provided additionally guidance in an opinion issued in *General Electric Co. v. Joiner*.[31] The *Joiner* ruling reaffirmed that a trial judge not only had the authority but also the responsibility to evaluate whether an expert's conclusions have been extrapolated from insufficient or inadequate data. Since most judges are not scientists, it was imperative for a party challenging the admissibility of expert testimony to be able to educate the court. Supreme Court Justice Breyer recommended in his concurring opinion in *Joiner* that parties provide the court with specially trained court appointed experts to assist the trial judge.

Unfortunately, this clarification of *Daubert* came too late to save Dow Corning from bankruptcy. The bankruptcy of Dow Corning, one of the largest manufacturers of the silicone gel breast implant, is a prime example of how the legal system disregarded the science and failed to impose standards regarding what scientific information could be (should be) considered admissible. Dow Corning filed for protection under Chapter 11 of the U.S. Bankruptcy Code on May 15, 1995, primarily due to the extensive litigation and the lack of support from their insurers. The company had been a named defendant in numerous class action lawsuits against several silicone gel breast implant manufacturers.

After Dow Corning filed for bankruptcy protection, other manufacturers of silicone gel breast implants tried to ease their own litigation burden. As a result of the negative publicity about implants and the subsequent litigation surrounding the controversy, most of the other implant manufacturers decided that the best business decision was to withdraw from the market.

Trying to consolidate supervision of the silicone gel breast implant cases nationwide, the Judicial Panel on Multi-District Litigation ordered all federal silicone gel breast implant cases to be transferred to U.S. District Judge Sam C. Pointer, Jr, of the federal court in Birmingham, Alabama, for coordination of all pretrial proceedings. The task of the scientific panel was to hear both sides of

**Table 9.3**
**Selected listing of breast implant trials and verdicts**

| Case (year) | Winner | Verdict |
|---|---|---|
| *Doe v. 3M* (1982) | Plaintiff | $25,000 |
| *Forbes v. Dow Corning* (1983) | Defense | 0 |
| *Brown v. 3M* (1984) | Plaintiff | $100,000 |
| *Stern v. Dow* (1984) | Plaintiff | $1.7 million (settled) |
| *Livshitz v. Natural Y Surgical Specialties* (1991) | Plaintiff | Remitted to $1.7 million then settled |
| *Phillips v. Baxter* (1991) | Defense | 0 |
| *Toole v. Baxter* (1991) | Plaintiff | Remitted to $2.7 million then settled |
| *Hopkins v. Dow Corning* (1991) | Plaintiff | $7.3 million |
| *Goldrich v. Natural Y Surgical Specialties* (1991) | Defense | 0 |
| *Craft v. McGhan* (1992) | Defense | 0 |
| *Johnson v. MEC* (1992) | Plaintiff | $25 million (settled) |
| *Turner v. Dow* (1993) | Defense | 0 |
| *Stevens, Mackenzie, Hudson v. Dow* (1995) | Plaintiff | $2.67 million |
| *Grimes v. Baxter* (1995) | Plaintiff | $400,000 (appealed) |
| *Valentine v. Baxter* (1995) | Mistrial | |
| *Bean, Newell, Habel v. Baxter* (1995) | Defense | 0 |
| *Kendrick and Surman v. Baxter* (1995) | Defense | 0 |
| *Mahlum v. Dow* (1995) | Plaintiff | $14.1 million (appealed) |
| *Morriss v. Surgitek* (1995) | Mistrial | |
| *Schilleci, Berry, Hammes and Hendricks v. Baxter* (1995) | Defense | 0 |
| *Gamblin v. 3M* (1995) | Mistrial | |
| *Jennings v. Baxter* (1996) | Defense | 0 |
| *Tyson v. 3M* (1996) | Defense | 0 |
| *Kelley v. Baxter* (1997) | Defense | 0 |
| *Atterbury, Bliven-Olson, Bonds and Stewart v. 3M* (1997) | Plaintiff | $1.5 million (reversed on appeal) |
| *Lescher and Wheeless v. Baxter* (1997) | Defense | 0 |
| *Duke v. 3M* (1997) | Plaintiff | $30,000 |
| *Stirling v. MEC* (1997) | Defense | 0 |

the issue, as well as to assess the scientific evidence presented in silicone gel breast implant cases. The establishment of a Delphi panel was an excellent step to help weed out the "junk science" that had been previously introduced and relied on in the courts. The panel of experts (immunologist, epidemiologist, toxicologist, and rheumatologist) was instructed to review and critique the scientific literature pertaining to the possibility of a causal association between silicone gel breast implants and disease. The report affirmed findings that were consistent with those reported in the British IRG study and the U.S. IOM evaluation: silicone gel breast implants were safe. The increased use of court appointed, neutral expert panels to advise judges on the scientific credibility of evidence, used by both the plaintiffs and the defense, was a positive step.[32]

In Oregon, U.S. District Court Judge Robert E. Jones, too, heard arguments on the scientific admissibility of evidence relative to alleged silicone breast implant-related diseases. Judge Jones formed four neutral panelists to advise on the admissibility of opinions offered by plaintiffs' experts pending in his jurisdiction. Judge Jones ruled that plaintiffs' "scientific" experts could not offer opinions on causation issues; their opinions were not based on tested hypotheses, and none of the studies cited showed an increase in relative risk greater than 2 for any disease. He ruled that their opinions differed from the prevailing consensus. His ruling, however, did not bind other federal district courts, but Judge Jones did demonstrate the appropriate use of a scientific advisory panel.

Despite the agreement among scientists that silicone gel breast implants were safe, the events that transpired prior to these panel reports still had to be handled. The cost of litigating was tremendous; it was estimated that the manufacturers were paying in excess of $1 million per litigated case in legal fees. Manufacturers wanted to resolve the issue and return to normal business operations. A Revised Settlement Program was established to provide a fund to compensate women who had health problems associated with silicone gel breast implants, saline-filled breast implants, and breast implants with polyurethane covering. Current and future claims for a fifteen-year period were to be reimbursed for medical diagnosis and evaluation, removal of the implants, removal of ruptured implant, and for specific autoimmune diseases. Women, of course, would have to meet the court's criteria, an important point given that numerous studies showed no link between silicone gel breast implants and disease.

## THE FDA'S ROLE

The FDA's role in the silicone gel breast implant saga is a significant one. Prior to 1976, medical devices essentially were unregulated. Manufacturers and patients determined safety, but this changed on May 28, 1976, when Congress passed the Medical Device Amendments Act. This act gave the FDA authority to regulate medical devices such as breast implants. The law requires manufacturers of new medical devices to show first that they are safe, effective, and properly labeled before the devices are allowed on the market. Rather than require products already on the market to undergo the rigorous studies newly required, the FDA simply "grandfathered" most of those into the new system. Since breast implants had been on the market for over ten years with a relatively positive safety record, these devices were among those for which new safety studies were not required. In 1982, the FDA proposed that breast implant manufacturers provide additional evidence on the safety of the product, but it was only in 1988 that the FDA mandated that the manufacturers provide such evidence. Oddly, this ruling was not enforced for implants until 1991.[33] Even with this mandate, only four of the thirty manufacturers submitted the required evidence.

In 1992, the FDA declared a temporary moratorium on the use of gel-filled silicone implants because there was new information available that raised questions about the product's safety. This new information consisted of Dow Corning's internal documents that a lawyer collected while investigating the company. These documents illustrate just how little the company knew about the safety of the product. One memo read, "Is there something in the implant that migrates out or off the mammary prostheses? Yes or no? Does it continue for the life of the implant or is it limited or controlled for a period of time? Does it come from the gel or the envelope or both? What is it?"[34]

Also in 1992, the FDA restricted the use of silicone gel breast implants to participants in clinical observational studies only conducted under the Investigational Device Exemptions (IDE) regulation or a FDA-approved adjunct study. The implants would be available only to women who needed reconstruction after mastectomy; women who wanted implants for breast augmentation would not be eligible to be enrolled in these studies.

The FDA's decision to ban silicone gel breast implants in the early 1990s probably stemmed from the belief that the agency had insufficient data on the safety and effectiveness of the device. Most of the epidemiological studies were not published until the mid- to late-1990s. During this same time period, there was intense political and public pressure to remove silicone gel implants from the market. The FDA Commissioner, Dr. David Kessler, was careful to note that the ban was implemented not because gel-filled implants had been shown to be unsafe, rather, because adequate data on their safety had not been provided to the FDA. The FDA's action perhaps heightened the image that breast implants are unsafe. Following the ban in 1992, there was a wave of multimillion-dollar lawsuits filed. It became apparent that some lawyers were trying to recruit women through advertisements in newspapers and then referred these women to doctors who would certify that the individual was afflicted by debilitating autoimmune diseases. The lawsuits culminated in a massive class action lawsuit that resulted in a $4 billion settlement award! This settlement was overturned, but the damage had been done.

In 2004, Inamed Corp, a breast implant manufacturer, asked the FDA to consider restoring silicone gel breast implants to the market. The FDA rejected the application and issued new guidelines delineating the information the manufacturer must provide documenting the safety and effectiveness of the device. The FDA needed information on a reasonable assurance of safety before further review of a premarket approval. Almost one year later, and thirteen years after most of the silicone gel breast implants were banned, the FDA, in a surprising turnaround, recommended allowing silicone gel breast implants to return to the U.S. market, but only under strict conditions that limit how easily women can get them. Mentor Corp, another implant manufacturer, persuaded the FDA that its newer silicone implants were reasonably safe and more durable compared with the older versions. ("Reasonably safe" was not defined by the FDA). However, the FDA ruled that the Inamed Corp again failed to satisfy lingering concerns about how often the implants break apart and leak. Mentor had performed more convincing research that the implants only rarely break, even though this research was based on a three-year follow up and on a few hundred women. While sales can resume, Mentor must meet strict conditions, including having individuals sign a consent form acknowledging implant risks. It was also recommended that women get an MRI scan five years after their implant is inserted and every two years thereafter.[35]

## ROLE OF THE MEDIA

The media's handling of the silicone gel breast implant controversy most certainly had a direct impact on public perception. In retrospect, a number of journalists and media organizations did not present a balanced and informed view on the safety of silicone implants. More often than not during the 1990s, media reports on the silicone implant story were inflammatory and not well balanced. As early as 1991, CBS refused to air a Dow Corning rebuttal to the rebroadcast of Connie Chung's show in which she implied that silicone gel breast implants were unsafe. It was only when the scientific studies began to show that implants were not a health risk that journalists began to write their stories in a different light. By the time that these articles were published, however, it was too late to undo the damage already done.

## THE RETURN OF SILICONE BREAST IMPLANTS

After a fifteen-year ban, the FDA, on November 18, 2006, announced its approval of the marketing of silicone gel breast implants, but with some strings attached. The implants were to be approved for use only for reconstruction surgery regardless of the age of the woman, and for augmentation in women ages 22 and older. For all women, however, regular magnetic resonance imaging screening would be required for early detection of implant rupture. The FDA also is requiring that the two California companies who make the implants (Allergan Corp.—formerly Inamed Corp.—of Irvine and Mentor Corp. of Santa Barbara) conduct a large postapproval study tracking 80,000 patients to make sure that no health concerns arise. Specifically, each device maker will be required to continue follow-up studies for ten years, conduct a focus group study of the patient labeling, continue laboratory studies to characterize types of device failure, and track each implant in the event that the medical profession and patients need to be notified of updated product information.[36]

In approving the return of silicone implants, the FDA did not mean to imply that the devices are risk-free. The FDA simply said that it had "reasonable assurance" that the devices were safe and effective. The devices are still prone to rupture, contracture, or to cause pain and inflammation in the breast. The FDA's decision was based on a thorough review of the device-makers clinical and preclinical studies, as well as an inspection of each company's manufacturing facilities to determine compliance with FDA's Good Manufacturing Practices (GMPs). The FDA has a good understanding of what complications can occur and at what rates. Given the FDA's poor track record in forcing companies to complete postmarketing studies, the agency will have to be extra careful in monitoring the risks of the device over time.

## LESSONS TO BE LEARNED

The scientific evidence almost uniformly suggested that women with silicone gel breast implants were not at a statistically increased risk for disease or for cancer. In fact, most women with such implants did not experience any serious complications. Yet, there were women who did experience complications and systemic illness and attributed these symptoms to their implant and vociferously voiced their views. Many who had broken implants did suffer disabling pain, but others did not. For many, the decision to have breast implants surgically inserted was a good one, for others, it was disastrous. Many sought legal redress through class action and individual lawsuits aided and abetted by plaintiff lawyers who tried to recover damages from the manufacturers for possible systemic diseases that their clients claimed had been "caused" by the implant.

In retrospect, the silicone gel breast implant litigation highlights the weaknesses in the legal system, the less than stellar handling of the case by the FDA, and the power of the media. Looking back, the escalation of the breast implant debate was fueled by plaintiff lawyers and by the misrepresentation of the body of scientific evidence by the media. It should be said that although the manufacturers agreed to settle the cases, that decision did not signify that silicone implants were harmful. The financial toll on the manufacturers was such that continuing the litigation would have been more harmful than paying out settlements.

The silicone gel breast implant story highlights the dangers of permitting unscientific studies to be introduced into the courts. Without proper scientific evidence, finding a party guilty or liable violates the spirit of the law and undermines the purpose of the legal system. However, as was evident in the early court cases, judges and juries often did not know what was considered valid testimony or valid scientific evidence. To ensure that the scientific evidence proffered was not based on personal opinions, the courts, over the years, have tried to set standards upon which expert testimony must be assessed. Weeding out "junk science" was a necessary first step. Only those studies that meet standards for scientific proof should be admissible in court, and this should be the norm for any tort case.

The silicone gel breast implant litigation example is a microcosm for so much that was wrong with the system. While there are many women who truly believe that they have been poisoned by their implants, there are many others who would disagree. One woman who received a silicone gel implant in 2001 was reported as saying, "We all deserve to feel beautiful, and if not beautiful, at least normal."[37] Yes, but both the individual and her physician should be aware of the potential risks of any medical device or product. Hopefully, the lessons learned from the implant litigation and the legal precedent set by the Daubert ruling will raise the standards of admissible evidence by mandating the use of scientifically sound epidemiological evidence in order to show elevated risk and causation.

# —— 10 ——

# Obesity and Public Policy

## with Joanna M. Paladino

> Despite the myths about Americans' self reliance, the U.S. government has
> a long tradition of intervening in private behavior.[1]

Americans are now the fattest people on earth. How Americans achieved this
dubious distinction can partially be understood by examining the economics and
politics of the food industry. Greg Critser's book, *Fat Land: How Americans
Became the Fattest People in the World,* clearly and concisely illustrates the
relationship between the government and the food industry and points an accus-
ing finger at both.[2] He argues that overproduction of food has led to overconsumption, and that getting fat is less an aberration than a normal response to the
American environment. "Supersizing" of portions has led to people eating much
more than they would otherwise. Human hunger is quite elastic, and people
presented with gigantic portions happily consume more. In just two decades,
Americans have learned to eat, on average, an additional 200 calories a day.

Obesity is now considered to be one of the most pressing medical and public
health issues, not just in the United States, but also in the world, affecting
children as well as adults. Just as the media routinely covers reports of famine
and malnutrition around the world, now obesity, at times referred to as an epidemic, makes front-page news. In the United States alone, more than half of
the population is tipping the scales at an unhealthy rate. Americans have been
getting heavier for three decades, and with this extra weight has come serious
medical consequences, not to mention the associated economic costs. Whether
counted in terms of the number of lives affected or by its costs, obesity is a
serious problem. Indeed, the numbers are shocking:

- 129.6 million adult Americans (64% of the population) are overweight or obese.
- 300,000 deaths a year can be linked to obesity.
- Obesity-related health care costs $117 billion a year.
- Americans spend $30 billion a year on weight-loss products and services.
- Obesity among children is increasing alarmingly.[3]

## BACKGROUND

Carrying excess weight was once a sign of health and prosperity. In many cultures, being heavy was associated with physical attractiveness, strength, and fertility. For example, obesity was also considered a symbol of wealth and social status in cultures prone to food shortages or famine. The Belgian painter Rubens (1577–1640), well known for his paintings of voluptuous, full female figures (the word *Rubenesque* refers to plumpness), captured the beauty of the full-figure. Roly-poly children and ample girths in men and women, however, were later on viewed in a less positive light. In the twentieth century, especially in Western cultures, the obese body shape became a symbol of unattractiveness and even gluttony. Hollywood glamorized thinness. Diet gurus proliferated (and prospered). A huge weight-loss industry was born. Being fat was no longer seen as a positive thing.

Until recently, obesity was not considered to be a major health or economic problem. Rather, it was an individual lifestyle problem with medical consequences for that individual. But, in 2001, almost 25 years after the National Institutes of Health (NIH) sounded the alarm on increasing obesity rates in America, the U.S. Surgeon General's "Call to Action" paper proclaimed that overweight and obesity have reached epidemic proportions.[4] And, in 2004, the U.S. Department of Health and Human Services officially classified obesity as a disease. Much of the problem lies not only with the overabundance and overproduction of food, but also the type of food being produced. Many countries, especially the wealthy ones, have much more food than they need. In the United States, for example, the food supply provides 3,800 kilocalories per person per day, which is twice as much as is required by many adults.[5] Yet, the agriculture, food product, restaurant, diet, and drug industries all profit by people eating more than is necessary, and the respective lobby groups certainly discourage the government from doing anything that would inhibit the production and marketing of food, healthy and nutritious or otherwise. Some believe that food marketing promotes weight gain, and certainly All You Can Eat buffets as well as the larger portions of food now served in many eating establishments do not help matters.[6] As the debate simmers about what to do about the increasing girth of Americans, the pharmaceutical industry is poised to capitalize on this huge market by developing and marketing drugs to "cure" obesity.

This chapter focuses on the causes and consequences of obesity, as well as the economics and politics associated with it. The main debate between "personal responsibility" and "public interest" is complex and contentious. Compounding the issue is that most people do not consider being fat a disease. They see overweight and obesity as a lifestyle problem. Many are confused by the changing food pyramid guidelines, the ever-changing list of foods to eat and not to eat, and celebrity diet crazes. Added to all this is the daily bombardment of advertisements for inexpensive and plentiful fast food options. The obesity epidemic has reached the point where even McDonald's, the purveyor of Big Macs and super-sized portions of French fries, is throwing its weight behind obesity research as well as the promotion of what it calls balanced, active lifestyles.

Given that the science is clear about the causes and correlates of overweight and obesity, what is the government's policy to help stem this epidemic? What are the economics and politics of obesity? What has been the food industry's response to the situation?

## QUANTIFYING OBESITY

One's body has 30 to 40 billion fat cells, and if one eats calories that one doesn't need for immediate energy, most of the excess is stored as fat. The body has an almost unlimited capacity to store fat. When food energy intake exceeds energy expenditure, fat cells take in the energy and store it as fat:

$$\text{net energy} = \text{energy intake} - \text{energy expenditure}$$

One can easily become overweight or obese from consuming more food energy than one expends in physical activity. There is a difference, however, between excess fat and excess weight. Being classified as overweight usually refers to a weight that is greater than what is considered healthy for an individual of certain age and height. An individual may be overweight but not be overfat; that is, athletes may be overweight because of a large body frame or muscle development, but they are not overfat. Weight alone, then, is not the best indicator of being overweight, but for the vast majority of obese individuals, chances are that if one is overweight, one is also overfat.

There are neurobiological mechanisms that are involved in the development and maintenance of obesity including the discovery of leptin receptors and other hormonal mechanisms that influence the regulation of appetite and food intake. Additionally, there are numerous environmental and behavioral factors that could lead to overweight and obesity:

- a sedentary lifestyle/physical inactivity; a high glycemic diet (a diet that consists of meals that give high postprandial blood sugar—foods and beverages with a high sugar content such as soft drinks, candy, and desserts are loaded with empty calories and provide few, if any, nutrients)
- eating disorders (binge eating disorders, for example)
- smoking cessation (some smokers gain weight after they give up cigarettes, but the benefits of stopping smoking usually outweighs the few extra pounds gained)

- genetic factors (genes influence the amount of body fat and fat distribution and can make one more susceptible to gaining weight)
- underlying illness (e.g., hypothyroidism)
- some medications (certain drugs such as corticosteroids, tricyclic antidepressants, insulin, and hormones may cause weight gain)
- private behavior—the overconsumption of food and drink

In addition to the above listed factors, one of the most frequently mentioned explanations for the huge increase in the number of overweight and obese individuals is proliferation of processed foods and fast food restaurants. Since 1980, for example, there has been a dramatic growth in the number of fast food outlets, and with the intense competition for market share came increased portion sizes. McDonald's, for example, increased its French fries portions from 200 calories in 1960 to over 600 calories today. Supersized portions not only at the fast food chains but also at other restaurant establishments have become the norm.

There are several ways to measure body fat; the most frequently used technique is the body mass index (BMI), a simple method for estimating body fat that was developed by the Belgian statistician and anthropometrist Adolphe Quetelet.[7] The BMI is calculated by dividing a person's weight in pounds by the square of height in inches multiplied by 703. A BMI of less than 18.5 is considered underweight; a BMI of 18.5 to 24.9 reflects normal weight; a BMI of 25 to 29.9 is considered to be overweight and an individual with a BMI of 30 to 39.9 is considered to be obese. The BMI, however, should not used as a sole clinical predictor of obesity because it does not take into account differing ratios of adipose (fat) to lean tissue, nor does it distinguish between differing forms of adiposity. In healthy adults, an acceptable level of body fat ranges from 18% to 23% in men and 25% to 30% in women. For children and adolescents who are growing, the Centers for Disease Control and Prevention (CDC) has created a BMI-for-age growth chart for both males and females, and children at or above the 95th percentile on the sex-specific chart are classified as overweight.[8] The BMI, however, does not take into account differences in body composition.

Another way to determine obesity is to assess percent body fat. The absolute waist circumference (>102 cm in men and >88 cm in women) or the waist–hip ratio (>0.9 for men and >0.85 for women) are used as measures of central obesity. Another way to measure body fat is to weigh a person underwater, but a simpler method is either the skinfold test, in which a pinch of skin is precisely measured to determine the thickness of the subcutaneous fat layer, or bioelectrical impedance analysis, which is a test usually carried out in specialty clinics.

## THE HEALTH EFFECTS OF OBESITY

There is a rich literature showing that being overweight in general, and obese in particular, is not healthy. Obesity is associated with increased mortality relative to individuals in the normal weight category. Depending on the methods of analysis, it is estimated that obesity is associated with between 111,000 and 325,000 excess deaths per year.[9,10] The evidence for the relationship between obesity and chronic illnesses is clear. Being obese, and to a certain extent being overweight, increases the risk of developing a whole host of lifestyle diseases. While diseases of the heart, cancers, and strokes are the top three causes of death in the United States, obesity is both an independent risk factor for coronary heart disease (CHD) and death from heart disease, as well as a risk factor for high blood pressure and elevated serum cholesterol.[11,12] Obesity has also been causally linked to a number of other diseases including vascular disease, diabetes mellitus, obstructive sleep apnea, liver disease, gall bladder disease, degenerative joint disease, osteoarthritis, and certain types of cancers. These conditions are often chronic and debilitating and may lead to diminished quality of life, increased dependence on the health care system, and increased work disability.[13,14]

The relationship between obesity and type II diabetes, in particular, has been publicized widely, primarily because of a large increase in the incidence of this disease within the past few years. It is now well known that the risk of type II diabetes increases with increasing BMI in both men and women.[15,16] Not only is absolute BMI a major predictor of the risk for diabetes mellitus, but changes in weight are associated with changes in diabetes risk as well. Women with a weight gain of eleven pounds or more were found to have a significantly increased risk of diabetes mellitus; moreover, women who lost at least eleven pounds reduced their risk of diabetes by as much as 50% or more.[17] Another study further quantified the risk, finding that weight gain over a period of ten years is associated with a substantial risk for diabetes—for every two-pound increase in weight, the risk for diabetes increases by 4.5%.[18]

The parallel obesity and diabetes epidemics reveal stark realities about the line between health and illness, a line that is influenced by genetics, race and ethnicity, and economics. The environment, too, influences the eating behavior of children and adolescents, as those who live in neighborhoods described as low income with high levels of poverty, low education, and low housing value are more likely to have poor dietary habits compared with those living in higher socioeconomic neighborhoods.[19] On a national level, the risk of diabetes is at least twice as great in Mexican Americans, Puerto Rican Americans, and non-Hispanic blacks than in non-Hispanic whites, and the prevalence of physician-diagnosed diabetes continues to rise most steeply among Mexican Americans and African Americans.[20]

The issue of ethnicity, obesity, and diabetes was poignantly addressed in a *New York Times* expose, "Living at an Epicenter of Diabetes, Defiance, and Despair" in January 2006.[21] In New York City, a line drawn across East 96th Street separates East Harlem to its north, a neighborhood with predominantly black and Latino residents with a median household income of $20,111, from the Upper East Side to its south, a neighborhood with predominantly White residents with a median household income of $74,446. The rates of obesity and diabetes are about *four* times and *sixteen* times greater, respectively, in East Harlem than in the Upper East Side neighborhood, and residents north of East 96th Street are about ten times more likely to be hospitalized because of diabetes and almost five times more likely to die because of their diabetes than residents south of East 96th Street.

The article highlights the neighborhood context in which residents of East Harlem live and depicts a world that is "hospitable" to obesity and diabetes. A study published in the *American Journal of Preventive Medicine* found that there are over three times as many supermarkets in wealthier neighborhoods than in lower income neighborhoods and four times as many in white neighborhoods than in black neighborhoods. Fast food restaurants and small corner grocery stores (bodegas) are also significantly more common in lower income neighborhoods, which suggests that in neighborhoods with fewer supermarkets or large chain stores there are limited options to buy healthy food because bodegas tend to stock less healthy food choices at generally higher prices.[22]

While inner-city, poorer communities tend to have higher rates of obesity and diseases related to obesity, on a state level, there are some interesting differences, which probably also reflect lifestyle and diet. A study conducted by the Trust for America's Health found that when using BMI to categorize weight, more than 20% of adults are obese in forty-three states and in the District of Columbia. Colorado is the slimmest state, with approximately 17% of adults categorized as obese and 36.1% as overweight. States in the northeast and West are the leanest, whereas nine of the ten fattest states are in the South. Mississippi is the fattest state, with 29.5% of adults considered to be obese and 36.4% overweight. Alabama was second with 28.7% of adults obese, and West Virginia was third at 28.6% adults obese. Thirty-one states had a higher percentage of dangerously overweight or obese adults in 2005 than in 2004. Obesity rates were little changed in eighteen states and the District of Columbia.[23] Those states with the highest percentage of obese and overweight individuals also had the highest rates of type II diabetes.

The situation has serious implications for the future. Unless things change dramatically, obesity will continue to be a major public health problem, primarily because overweight and obese children have an increased risk of becoming overweight or obese adults. The implications of excess weight between childhood and adulthood have been documented in numerous studies over the years.[24–26] Although the information about type II diabetes in children is limited, data that have been collected on children in specific populations clearly show an alarming picture. Although type II diabetes is still considered to be rare in childhood, certain cohorts, such as Pima Indians living in Central Arizona and Mexican and Hispanic children in general, have been shown to have a very high prevalence of type II diabetes. In fact, overall, the prevalence of type II diabetes among ten- to nineteen-year-olds in America has significantly increased over the last thirty years, reflecting the concomitant increase in weight among children. In Cincinnati, Ohio, for example, the incidence of type II diabetes among adolescents ten to nineteen years of age has increased more than tenfold, from 0.7 per 100,000 persons in 1982 to 7.2 per 100,000 persons in 1994.[27] Obesity was found to be a strong risk factor for and predictor of type II diabetes among these children, along with family history. One in five children diagnosed with type II diabetes in this study had at least one additional obesity-related condition.

The numbers are staggering, and the implications for the future health of so many in the population are scary. Over a period of two decades, the prevalence of obesity has doubled for adults, and the number of overweight children has nearly tripled.[28,29] From 2003–2004, 17.1% of the children and adolescents aged two to nineteen years were classified as being overweight, and 32.2% of adults aged twenty and older were classified as being obese.[30] Even being a little overweight is not necessarily a good thing. A recent study examined the living habits of more than 527,000 men and women aged fifty to seventy-one and found that those who were overweight at age fifty had a 20% to 40% higher risk of death than healthy weight individuals, and those who were obese had a 100% to 200% higher risk of premature death.[31] It was well-known that being obese (thirty or more pounds over a healthy weight) increased the risk of premature death, but this large-scale study shows that even being a little overweight also increases the chances of premature death. If the trend continues, if we do not effectively change the unhealthy, sedentary lifestyle that seems to permeate society, the burden of providing medical care, and paying for health care, will be significant.

## THE ECONOMICS OF FOOD

There were substantial changes in the quantity and variety of foods in the U.S. food supply over the decades, with much of the change due to advances in technology and alterations in marketing practices.[32] Historically, especially during the 1930s and 1940s, the addition of nutrients to foods through enrichment and fortification was an effective way to maintain and improve the overall nutritional quality of the food supply. By the 1950s, enrichment and fortification of foods, such as fortification of salt with iodine; fortification of milk with vitamin D; and enrichment of flour and grains with thiamin, riboflavin, niacin, and iron helped bring more healthy foods into the food supply. Production techniques and marketing changes also have been responsive to and reflective of dietary recommendations for fat, saturated fat, and cholesterol. But adherence with dietary recommendations is often slow and not easily achieved by the general population. Although Americans have made some positive dietary changes in terms of consumption of grain products, vegetables, and fruits, as well as the selection of lower fat animal foods from the dairy and meat groups, they are doing less well with overall consumption of sugars and sweeteners, total fat, and salt intake.

There is a common belief that people get fat because they eat too many car-bohydrates and sugars. The idea is that a high-carbohydrate diet leads to weight gain, higher insulin and blood glucose levels, and diabetes. Evidence now clearly shows that consumption of sugar-sweetened beverages, in particu-lar the carbonated soft drinks, are a key contributor to the epidemic of over-weight and obesity.[33] Sugar-sweetened beverages, especially soda, provide little nutritional benefit and increase the risk of obesity-related diseases such as diabetes. Nondiet soft drinks account for 47% of total added sugars in the diet.[34] Concomitant with the consumption of sodas is the increased intake of fruit drinks and fruitades (drinks made by adding water to powder or crystals), which are sweetened and consumed primarily by children. Consumption of these fruit drinks represents nearly 81% of the increase in caloric sweetener intake.[35] Therefore, it is not surprising to learn that consumption of carbohy-drates, largely in the form of added sugars, has increased dramatically,[36] which has prompted the call for individuals to choose beverages and foods that would decrease their intake of added sugars.[37,38]

In addition to the call to limit consumption of sugar in the diet, reduction of fat in the diet also has been advocated. Low-fat diets have been touted as a way to reduce weight and stay healthy, but do they really work? Findings from a large eight-year trial on women found that a low-fat diet did not cut health risks, and the results did not justify recommending low-fat diets to the public to reduce their heart disease or cancer risk![39] Women who were assigned to a low-fat diet (diet that had just 20% of its calories as fat) had the same rates of breast and colon cancer, heart attacks, and strokes as those women who ate whatever they pleased.

Before one accepts these findings as the gospel, it is important to understand that the diets of the two groups really did not differ all that much. Those who were on the low-fat diet cut calories from fat only by 8.2% compared with 1.1% in the other group. Also, the low-fat diet was not easy to follow. Most women in the low-fat diet were unable to maintain a diet with 20% of its calo-ries as fat. So, in all probability, a low-fat diet alone is not the magic bullet.

Scientists now know that the type of fat is actually very important, more so than the amount of fat consumed. Focusing just on total fat intake, without studying the different effects of different types of fat, is not helpful. Nonsatu-rated fats, such as those in olive oil, or omega-3 fats found in fish, for example, are healthier than saturated fat found in butter and beef. Trans fats, which are created by adding hydrogen to natural fat, are absolutely the worst type of fat. Trans fats have been linked with increased risks of heart disease and should be avoided if possible. The food industry only recently agreed to reduce or elimi-nate trans fat from most products.

Although sugar and sweeteners and certain types of fat in the diet have been on the food hit list, the daily consumption of salt (sodium) has soared and is now the target for reduced consumption. It has been known for decades that sodium consumption can lead to salt-induced high blood pressure and is a significant contributor to heart disease and stroke. Salt is ubiquitous in the American food supply being sprinkled on bread, cheese, soups, breakfast cereals, and just about everything else. Three-quarters of the salt consumed comes from processed foods, not from the salt shaker. Frozen foods, in particular, are loaded with sodium; a Hungry Man dinner, for example, has as many as 2,230 milligrams of sodium per serving, which is far more than the government's recommended daily allowance (less than 2,300 milligrams of sodium a day and the threshold should be 1,500 milligrams for certain individuals). On average, Americans consume more than 3,300 milligrams of sodium a day.

In an effort to draw attention to the persistently high level of salt in many processed foods, the American Medical Association (AMA) is mounting a campaign to have the food industry reduce sodium levels in foods. Interestingly, the AMA has never called for regulation of a food ingredient, but is now asking the Food and Drug Administration (FDA) to regulate salt as a food additive. Packaged food companies would then have to adhere to limits on allowable sodium levels for various categories of foods. Not surprisingly, the Salt Institute has begun its lobbying against salt regulation. (The total value of the salt market in the United States is $340 million.[40]) To date, the FDA has done little to focus on the issue, even though it is estimated that 150,000 lives could be saved annually if sodium levels in foods were cut in half.[41]

In the case of obesity, maybe focusing on the food industry in general is not so misguided. Food companies, as well as the government, are well aware of the economic implications of reversing the obesity epidemic. U.S. Department of Agriculture (USDA) economists have calculated that large adjustments would occur in the agriculture and processed food industries if people ate more healthfully.[42] Indeed, the primary sources of fat in the American diet are red meat, plant oils, and dairy products, and the government heavily subsidizes the producers of all three. Farm subsidies, too, often work against more healthful eating. How ironic is it that the federal agency in charge of national nutrition policy, the USDA, is caught in such a catch-22. As such, the government's action remains more focused on food purity and food labeling than on promoting nutritional value.

Although federal and state governments are responsible for the regulation, production, distribution, and consumption of food, no regulations exist to control the production or consumption of low-nutrition, high-fat foods. Pathetically, dietary fat in government-approved school lunches, for example, far exceeds recommended guidelines.[43] In fact, even though the link between diet and health outcomes is well established, and even with the medical profession's consensus about the dangers of being overweight, there has been little political effect. The federal government did not officially acknowledge the connection between diet and the risk of chronic disease until 1969 when a White House conference was held on food, nutrition, and health. Long after the medical profession, public interest groups, and even insurance companies warned about rising obesity, the federal government (finally) in 1977 began focusing on dietary guidelines. The focus was on fat consumption and the link between a high-fat, low-nutrition diet to cancer and heart disease.[44] But, federal enthusiasm as measured in budgetary allocations, was, and remains, limited.

Another factor that promotes overconsumption of food is readily available, plentiful, cheap, energy-dense foods. The United States is an economically driven society. Many of our choices come down to incentive, and food choice is no exception. By using an economic framework to analyze eating behaviors, economists have concluded that an individual will consume food within their budget that maximizes benefits such as taste and health and minimizes costs such as financial burden or losing health.[45] Preferences vary on an individual level—long-term health may not be important to some while weight gain may be a serious cost to others.

From a population standpoint, with such variations in preference, changing food pricing may have an impact on individual eating behaviors.[46] Price reductions on low-fat vending machine snacks, for example, significantly increased the sales of such items in both adults and adolescents.[47] In fact, a small study involving two high school cafeterias found that a 50% price reduction of fruits and carrots was effective in significantly raising the sales of these healthy foods.[48]

Factors that promote overconsumption, including the growth of the fast food industry, increasing portion sizes, and the marketing of high-calorie and highly sweetened snack foods, are clearly having a negative effect both on an individual and societal level.[49] How does all this contribute to overeating? According to nutrition expert Dr. Marion Nestle, food companies compete through expansive marketing campaigns, more often than not directed toward children, and promote larger portion sizes, thus fueling the American notion of getting more for less.[50] For example, in recent years, the sale of the 20-ounce bottle of soda has replaced the 12-ounce can as the standard in vending machines and convenience stores around the country.[51]

On an individual level, a person presented with a larger portion size often consumes it, which leads to an increase in caloric intake. One small study found that subjects consumed 30% more energy when faced with a larger portion size compared with a smaller one.[52] Industry markets a greater portion size, and the American public consumes it: a banner outside a McDonald's restaurant proclaims, "$1 Menu." Burger King advertises a "New Enormous Omelet Sandwich. It's Huge." At KFC, a sign boasted, "Feed Your Family for Under $4 Each." The industry profits by continuing to offer more for less, and the American public puts on weight and grows fatter.

It is often easier to blame someone else, to find a scapegoat, rather than take the more difficult route of taking action oneself. Blaming the food industry seems to be a knee-jerk reaction to the situation. According to Morone and Kersh, one of the key elements to an emerging political movement in response to a public health problem is "demonizing the industry."[53] With regard to the obesity epidemic, the fast-food industry is the target, and the American public the victims. With the publication of Eric Schlosser's book, *Fast Food Nation,* which is highly critical of the fast food industry and is being made into a film; with the 2004 release of the movie, "Super Size Me"; and with high-profile class action lawsuits against McDonald's, the public is increasingly exposed to the argument that the fast food industry is making us fat.[54] Perhaps in an effort to clean its image, perhaps because they really care, McDonald's, the world's biggest fast food company, has donated $2 million to the La Jolla, California-based Scripps Institute to fund research and programs aimed at preventing childhood obesity.[55] McDonald's marketing and advertising has indeed changed to reflect a more healthy way to eat, but will people who purchase their food from this chain go for the healthy salads or stick with the burger and fries? At least McDonald's is trying to move in the right direction.

## PUBLIC OPINION, MAGIC BULLETS, AND MESSAGES

How has the public reacted? Do they care? Are they doing anything to stem the battle of the bulge? In 2001, J. Oliver and T. Lee collected data about public opinion regarding obesity. It was thought that those individuals who consider obesity to be a serious health threat would more likely accept and support obesity-related policies.[56] According to the poll, Americans rank obesity behind cancer, AIDS, heart disease, and diabetes as a serious health concern, and although about half of the subjects were overweight, less than one-fourth of the respondents viewed their body weight as a serious health concern. When asked about factors contributing to obesity, 65% of respondents attributed obesity to an individual's lack of willpower to diet and exercise, although more than half also agreed that unhealthy food in restaurants and ineffective diets are to blame as well. The poll also revealed that Americans are less likely to support obesity-related policies than other public health regulations: 65% percent favor taxing cigarettes, whereas only 33% percent agree with a proposal to tax snack foods to subsidize the distribution of more healthful foods.

There is no doubt that Americans are getting the message to lose weight. It is difficult to surf the Web or watch the news without hearing about a new diet or a new product that promotes weight loss, often making it seem very simple. With over two-thirds of the population trying to lose or maintain weight, it is no wonder that consumers spend $33 billion per year on weight-loss efforts including low calorie foods, artificially sweetened products, and dieting books, plus an estimated $1–2 billion for weight-loss programs.[57] Despite this spending, the outcomes are somewhat discouraging regarding long-term weight control. A systematic review of the literature revealed that with patients using low-carbohydrate weight-loss strategies, weight reduction was primarily due to decreased calorie intake and increased diet duration rather than the reduction in carbohydrate intake.[58] The finding that weight loss primarily occurs when calories are reduced underscores the need to send a more consistent message to the American public, as many dieters opt for fat or carbohydrate reduction without calorie reduction.

Most studies show that even if weight loss is realized, keeping it off is another matter. One trial found that the Atkins diet produced more weight loss in obese patients than a high-carbohydrate, low-fat diet in the first six months, but the differences did not persist at one year due to more significant weight regain in the group of subjects using the Atkins diet.[59] The high attrition rate among participants in both diet programs in the aforementioned study emphasizes the difficulties in dieting and the need for long-term effective weight management. In a study of four popular diets, Atkins, Zone, Weight Watchers, and Ornish, all four diets produced a statistically significant yet modest decrease in weight at one year, yet in each diet group, only about one-quarter of the participants maintained a one-year weight loss of more than 5% of initial body weight.[60] Although there was a strong association between dietary adherence and weight loss, the study concluded that not one of the four popular diets produced adequate adherence rates.

## METABOLIC SYNDROME: IS IT A DISEASE?

The latest twist in the obesity debate is the attempt to transform obesity into a disease. Once something is classified as a disease, a disease classification code can be assigned, health insurers will reimburse providers for providing treatment, and pharmaceutical companies can develop drugs to "cure" the disease. The pharmaceutical companies have viewed obesity as the ultimate growth market. They have spent millions of dollars developing scores of drugs to treat obesity, and have been lobbying the FDA to make it easier to get obesity drugs to market. Although the FDA is still evaluating standards for developing obesity drugs, a new "disease" has been coined, which may make the pharmaceutical companies dreams come true: metabolic syndrome.

Metabolic syndrome, only concretely defined five years ago, is characterized by five risk factors: high blood pressure, high blood sugar, high triglycerides, low HDL ("good") cholesterol, and obesity. The World Health Organization (WHO) assigned it an International Classification of Disease code, which is important because it lets physicians diagnose and refer to it for insurance purposes. In reality, metabolic syndrome is analogous to obesity, as 85% of these individuals who have been labeled or diagnosed as having metabolic syndrome are obese or overweight.[61]

Many clinicians and most of the pharmaceutical companies view metabolic syndrome as the blockbuster disease of the twenty-first century. The metabolic syndrome market could be as big as $18 billion annually and has the potential to be bigger than the statin market for lowering cholesterol! The focus on drug therapy to treat the syndrome is a boon to the drug industry, which has more than 350 obesity and metabolic drugs in the pipeline. Acomplia (Rimonabant; Sanofi Pharmaceuticals) is the first of the metabolic syndrome drugs, and its sales could hit $5 billion a year.[62] The drug doesn't just promote weight loss, it improves HDL cholesterol and reduces insulin resistance. There are serious and unfortunate side effects such as depression and moodiness that are of concern but that is not stopping Sanofi, who has been working on this for twenty years, from heavily marketing the product. The drug is currently available in Europe.

There is no magic bullet for losing weight, but that does not deter the pharmaceutical industry for marketing its products. At this moment, there are two main drug classes that are approved by the FDA for the treatment of obesity in the United States: (1) inhibitors of fat absorption in the digestive system; that is, Orlistat (Xenical; Roche Pharmaceutical) inhibits fat digestion and excretes all undigested fat, and (2) medications that act on central nervous system neurotransmitters to suppress appetite, increase satiety, or increase thermogenesis; that is, Meridia (Sibutramine; Abbott Pharmaceutical) is the only appetite suppressing drug approved by the FDA.

Although there have been randomized, placebo-controlled trials demonstrating the efficacy of Orlistat compared with placebo in weight management for adults and adolescents, especially reports of significantly less weight *regain* after initial weight loss, a few questions remain.[63,64] These drugs will likely be prescribed to patients for the treatment of obesity, but would the drug be as effective in weight management without concomitant diet or exercise? One study found that the combination of group lifestyle-modification counseling and pharmacotherapy resulted in an average weight loss that was double that of the groups receiving either sibutramine alone or lifestyle modification alone.[65]

Yet, there are additional public health questions regarding pharmacotherapy and obesity treatment that remain unanswered. Many of the studies assess the efficacy of these drugs over a period of one year, or at most two years, and although they may measure weight loss and physiologic risk factors such as blood glucose and cholesterol, they do not measure the drug's effect on outcomes that are the actual concerns of the public, such as the development of type II diabetes, osteoarthritis, obstructive sleep apnea, or coronary heart disease.

In summary, there is limited information on effectiveness and sustainability of weight-loss drugs, although there is a potentially huge market for such therapy. While it may be easier to take a pill to lose weight, in reality, the side effects can be uncomfortable (see Table 10.1). Nevertheless, the pharmaceutical industry is spending huge amounts of money on marketing such drugs.

## THE POLITICS OF FOOD: THE GOVERNMENT'S ROLE

As the obesity epidemic grows, policymakers are trying to pursue legislative solutions modeled after the antismoking campaigns of the past. On a federal level, there appears to be little action, maybe because of the food industry's

**Table 10.1.**
**Types of weight-loss drugs**

| | |
|---|---|
| Amphetamines | Amphetamine-like appetite suppressants have been prescribed for weight loss. These types of drugs are very effective at curbing appetites and cause weight loss, but they are also highly addictive and can lead to overdoses. The drugs phentermine and fenfluramine (Wyeth-Ayerst Laboratories) were used in combination as part of the combination known as phen-fen. Phen-fen was approved for weight loss in 1996, but one year later was pulled from the market because of higher than expected risks of heart valve disease and pulmonary hypertension. |
| Monoamine (serotonin and norepinephrine) reuptake inhibitors | Anti-obesity drugs in this category work to suppress appetite. Sibutramine (Meridia; Knoll Pharmaceutical Company), approved for use in 1997, is thought to work by increasing the activity of certain chemicals, called norepinephrine and serotonin, in the brain. The drug boosts serotonin levels in the brain making users feel full. This drug is approved for use only in people who are very overweight. The drug's serious side effects include increased blood pressure and pulse rate, as well as an elevated risk of coronary artery disease. |
| Lipase inhibitors | This drug works in the intestines, where it blocks some of the fat from being absorbed and digested. The undigested fat is removed in bowel movements. The drug Orlistat (Xenical; Roche US Pharmaceuticals) was approved in 1999, and weight loss results have been shown. Some users, however, report flatulence and loose bowel movements making it unpopular among some patients. |
| CB1 cannabinoid receptor antagonist | This anti-obesity drug reduces appetite. Rimonabant (sold in the United Kingdom under the trade name Acomplia; Sanofi-Aventis) has not been approved by the FDA as of yet. While hailed as an effective weight loss drug, the side effects, including depression, anxiety, and irritability, have delayed a decision by the FDA. |

significant influence on policy. Perhaps fearing that they would be hit with huge judgments from lawsuits, the food industry is waging an aggressive campaign to make it very difficult for anyone to sue them successfully for causing obesity or obesity-related health problems. Lobbyists for food companies and restaurants help write legislation both on a state and federal level. These efforts have paid off for the industry. For example, on March 10, 2004, the House of Representatives voted 276–139 to ban "frivolous" lawsuits against the food industry (producers and sellers of food and nonalcoholic drinks) for making people fat; that is, for "claims of injury relating to a person's weight gain, obesity, or any health condition associated with weight gain or obesity."[66] The legislation, known as the "cheeseburger bill," was in response to lawsuits filed against the fast food industry. Supporters of the bill said that consumers couldn't blame others for the consequences of their actions, whereas opponents argued that the courts, not Congress, should determine when "obesity lawsuits" were frivolous. Other Congressional efforts have focused on trying to block attempts to tax snack foods and soft drinks.

In addition to passing laws most favorable to the food industry, the U.S. government also took aim at the WHO's dietary guidelines designed to curb the rising global epidemic of obesity and disease. In 2004, the U.S. Department of Health and Human Services publicly disputed some of the scientific evidence underlying the WHO's proposal for reducing obesity. Whereas WHO recommended that governments act on television advertising to children and urged individuals to cut down on fats and sugars in their diet, the United States favored dietary guidance that focused on the total diet, not just sugar and fat, as well as personal responsibility to choose a diet.[67] Critics said that the U.S. position favored the food industry trade groups and that the Bush administration was putting the interests of the junk food industry ahead of the health of people. Other governments, including the British government, were supportive of the global strategy promoted by WHO.

As is often the case, federal inaction has led to state action. State lawmakers have filed more than 140 bills aimed at obesity. Twenty states have enacted versions of a "commonsense consumption" law, which essentially prevents lawsuits seeking personal injury damages related to obesity from being tried. Eleven states have similar legislation pending. Adoption of the commonsense consumption laws shows how an organized and effective lobbying effort and a receptive legislative climate can shield food companies from court action. The food industry stands firmly against efforts to make food or restaurant companies legally accountable for the obesity problem. They maintain that it is each individual's "personal responsibility" to eat less, eat more healthy foods, and deal with his or her own weight problem.

In the District of Columbia and several states, lawmakers have debated bills that would require fast food and chain restaurants to post nutrition information such as caloric, fat, and sugar content on the menus. Twenty-five states are considering restrictions on the sale of soda and candy in schools, following successful efforts in Arkansas and Texas.[68] Three regulatory strategies have been tried: controlling the conditions of sale (especially those aimed at children), raising prices through taxes, and regulating marketing and advertising.[69] Ordinarily there is an exemption of food from the state sales tax, but statewide initiatives to tax junk foods are gaining popularity. Nineteen states tax junk foods that are considered not nutritious, such as candy and soft drinks. Most of the monies derived from the taxes, totaling about $1 billion per year, end up in the general treasury funds of the respective states, yet *none* of these funds are used specifically to promote nutrition programs![70] Meanwhile, it is not known whether these efforts actually affect the sales or consumption of the taxed foods, so the question remains: are these taxes actually leading to decreased consumption of junk food? If not, would the tax funds be useful if they fueled obesity prevention programs?

Food industry lobby groups have been somewhat successful in halting regulatory progression. About twelve cities or states have repealed portions of their snack and soft drink taxes in recent years because of strong lobbying from the food industry. In Ohio, for example, a tax of $0.008 per ounce of carbonated beverage and $0.64 per gallon of syrup, which generated about $59 million in revenue for the state, was repealed one year after it was enacted after the soft drink industry launched a campaign resulting in the addition of a constitutional amendment to repeal the tax to the ballot.[71] A 5% tax on snack food in Maryland was repealed in 1997 after Frito-Lay threatened not to build a plant in the state if the tax was not repealed. In addition to local and statewide lobbying, it is in the best interest of the food industry at all levels, including agriculture, food products, fast food, and restaurants, to capitalize on the amount of food people eat—and it follows naturally that food producers contribute large sums of money to congressional campaigns to ensure that the benefits continue.

Other regulatory strategies address the restriction of advertising and marketing of unhealthy foods, especially to children. Polls show that Americans are willing to support the regulation of advertising to children and the elimination of junk food in schools: 47% support the elimination of junk food in schools, and 57% support the regulation of advertisements directed at children.[72] Two states, Indiana and Massachusetts, have recently begun to address advertising to children, with one initiative that prohibits school boards from signing contracts with soda companies without public input and another that prohibits the use of soda advertisements on school buses.[73] Recently, attention is being focused on improving children's diet, especially what is served in the school lunchroom.

## HISTORY OF THE SCHOOL LUNCH PROGRAM

The CDC predicted that 30% to 40% of today's children would develop diabetes in their lifetimes if the current trend in overweight and obesity continues. When it comes to childhood obesity, personal responsibility really means parental responsibility. A survey conducted by the Public Agenda in 2002 found that 68% of American parents said that it was "absolutely essential" to teach their children good eating habits, but only 40% believed that they had succeeded.[74] Efforts to address this ticking time bomb of childhood obesity have focused on the school lunch program. The National School Lunch Act of 1946 guaranteed a hot lunch for every schoolchild who could not afford one. Ironically, this act was passed primarily because so many children at the time were too thin. The School Lunch Act put the federal government in the school food supply business, buying surplus products from farmers and sending these products along to the schools. The Johnson administration added free and reduced-cost breakfast, but this was pared back during the Reagan administration, the same administration that called catsup a vegetable. Under the Clinton administration, limits were set on fat at 30% of calories in a weekly menu. Today, 20% of the foods served in school cafeterias are USDA commodities. The government reimburses schools between 23 cents and $2.40 a meal, and requires every school to at least break even. Trying to introduce healthier foods into the school lunch program is not easy, as these products tend to cost more than the less nutritious foods.

The USDA's current definition of foods of minimal nutritional value focuses on whether a food has at least minimal amounts of one of eight nutrients; however, the definition does not address calories, saturated or trans fat, salt, or added sugars. USDA's standards apply only to food sold in the cafeteria, yet today vending machines in the schools have proliferated (83% of elementary schools, 97% of middle schools, and 99% of high schools sell food out of vending machines).[75] Not surprisingly, the majority of food/snacks and drinks sold in the vending machines are of poor nutritional quality. Tom Harkin (D-IA), a leader in trying to get bipartisan support for healthier school foods, described junk food sales in schools as being out of control and undercutting the school meal program. This situation provided the impetus for Senator Harkin and others to sponsor legislation to address this issue.

The Child Nutrition Promotion and School Lunch Protection Act of 2006 was introduced by a bipartisan group in Congress on April 6, 2006, in an effort to update USDA nutrition standards so that they conform with current nutrition science.[76] The act states that for a school food service program to receive federal reimbursements, school meals served by that program must meet science-based nutritional standards established by Congress and the Secretary of Agriculture. School meals must meet nutrition standards (limits on fat and saturated fat, for example). The act broadens the scope of the law to include all food sold on a school campus, such as vending machines, school stores, and snack bars.

Do such initiatives work? There have been numerous studies to measure the impact of school-based interventions. One such study, a randomized trial with the primary goal of reducing average percentage body fat in American Indian children, focused on a population particularly affected by rising overweight and obesity rates.[77] The intervention included a reduction in the fat content of school meals, three 30-minute physical activity sessions per week, classroom curricula focusing on healthy lifestyle choices, and family involvement. The study, however, found no significant reduction in body fat among intervention students compared with control students, although a significant reduction in the percentage of energy intake from fat and total energy intake as well as positive changes in knowledge and attitudes about nutrition were measured.

Multiple studies with varying levels of intervention components have resulted in variable degrees of increased physical activity in schools, reduced dietary fat intake, and increased intake of healthier foods such as fruits and vegetables.[78–80] Yet, most of the aforementioned studies either did not assess changes in body weight or percent body fat or found no difference in body weight or percent body fat between intervention and control groups. The one study that demonstrated a reduced prevalence of obesity among sixth- and seventh-grade girls employed an intervention with focused classroom sessions on decreased television viewing, increased fruit and vegetable consumption, decreased high-fat food consumption, and increased physical activity, and the outcome was primarily due to a reduction in television viewing![81] Similarly, a randomized, controlled trial found that a school-based intervention aimed at reducing television and video game use led to a significant relative decrease in the BMI of those children participating in the intervention, which was successful in that those children reported significantly less television viewing, video game use, and meals eaten while watching television.[82]

A recent effort to provide more nutritious food in the schools is sponsored by Dr. Arthur Agatston, the creator of the South Beach Diet. Elementary schools in Kissimmee, Florida, are part of the Healthier Options for Public Schoolchildren (HOPS) program designed to introduce nutritional change among primary school children.[83] While admirable in its scope and intent, evidence shows that the children did not lose weight nor was there significant change in BMI. The problem is that the program had no control over what the kids were eating outside of the school. Many other studies too failed to show a change in BMI. Long-term outcomes are not known because the students have not been followed prospectively.

Nevertheless, efforts continue. A report by Netscan's Health Policy Tracking Service described the state legislative school-based initiatives regarding nutrition and physical education.[84] One intervention that is gaining popular support is known as the "BMI Report Card." The practice of reporting students' body mass scores to parents originated a few years ago as just one tactic in a war on childhood obesity that would be coupled with the offering of fresh, low-fat foods in the cafeteria. Arkansas, in an initiative spearheaded by governor Mike Huckabee who recently lost over one hundred pounds himself, was the first to pass a law in 2003 requiring that schools calculate the BMI of students yearly and include that number on report cards that are sent home to parents along with information about changes in lifestyle that promote healthy eating and increased physical activity. Illinois, New York, Pennsylvania, Tennessee, and West Virginia have also passed legislation requiring that public schools monitor student BMIs.

Critics of the BMI report card feel that this could demoralize a student and could result in eating disorders and social stigma. The BMI is not necessarily an accurate indication of overweight or obesity. Perhaps positive results could be achieved by limiting the amount of junk food, improving the nutritional content of the food served, and increasing the number of hours for gym class.

Along the line of this thinking, thirty-two states are currently considering legislation to establish or amend nutritional standards in schools. In Arizona, for example, lawmakers passed a bill prohibiting sugary, carbonated beverages from being sold in elementary and middle schools.

Although there have been many other state legislative initiatives in schools, such as raising nutrition education requirements and funding, outreach to parents, restrictions on vending machines, and nutritional standards for cafeteria meals, the greatest number of legislative proposals introduced and enacted are directed at increasing physical education requirements and funding in schools. Twenty-eight states are currently considering bills that set standards on physical activity, physical education, and health education with regard to physical fitness.[85] In Maryland, for example, the Student Health and Fitness Act of 2006, which passed the Senate but awaits a House committee, would mandate that all students in grades kindergarten through five receive sixty minutes of physical education per week that would gradually increase to 150 minutes per week over the course of schooling, along with baseline and annual physical fitness assessments.

## WHERE DO WE GO FROM HERE?

Although knowledge of the increasing importance of diet and exercise in health maintenance and disease prevention is growing, we live in a society that encourages a lifestyle that is not optimal for the achievement of either. It is true that something needs to be done to combat the obesity epidemic. Certainly, emphasis on public education and the development of public health strategies is a start. Support for regulatory and legal actions at the local, state, and federal levels is important. The goal should be not to take away personal choice, but to create an environment in which an individual may make a *better* choice. With regard to obesity, this concept is even more complex because there is no equivalent to "Don't Smoke" or "Just Say No to Drugs." The issue is not how social and environmental change can occur in the current political climate, but how politics in the future (public policy) can contribute to social and environmental change.

The simple message to eat five servings of fruit and vegetables per day to stay healthy and fit is probably simplistic and unworkable. Every day individuals are bombarded by contradictory and confusing messages about weight loss and health. The government's frequent changes to the food pyramid, for example, send confusing and conflicting messages. How many servings of what foods do I really need for a healthy diet? The United States is a "headline" society, thriving on quick and convenient messages. In fact, it has been shown that consumers may not process information at a certain level of complexity, so the lack of information about effective weight management requires a solution that does not necessarily provide *more* information but rather provides a clear, simple, and efficacious message that can be processed easily by the American public. Confounding the issue is the fact that many Americans just do not view overweight and obesity as being a serious problem. Certainly most would like to lose weight, but actually doing so requires a discipline and focus that many do not have. It is much easier to take a pill to reduce one's cholesterol or high blood pressure than it is to live a healthier lifestyle. With the slew of anti-obesity drugs poised to hit the market, many might view taking a pill as the most efficient means of losing weight. But pharmaceuticals can do only so much; without lifestyle changes and changes in diet, long-term results will be hard to sustain.

As confusion typifies anti-obesity policies, Americans are getting fatter. It is one thing to consider mandating nutrition labels on menus, or improving school lunch programs, or even imposing taxes on high-calorie, low-nutrition foods, but what would probably be a better tactic is to regulate the food and drink industry to ensure that the foods produced are nutritionally in line with existing guidelines and regulations. Reducing the use of saturated and trans fats in food products, for example, reducing the sodium content in prepared foods, and encouraging the consumption of fruits, vegetables, and fiber, would be a good start to help people eat a more healthy diet. Subsequent efforts could then focus on helping those who lead unhealthy lives to begin to do their part in fighting the obesity epidemic. The battle cannot be won without all parties working together.

# ——11——

# Disease Prevention through Vaccination: The Science and the Controversy

## with Tony Rosen, MPH

I shall never have smallpox for I have had cowpox. I shall never have an ugly pockmarked face.[1]

## INTRODUCTION

Each one of us is constantly warding off the potential for infection or disease. After all, the world is filled with countless microbes, fortunately most of which are harmless and some even beneficial. But, there are plenty of microbes that can hurt us (pathogens, from the Greek word for disease, "pathos"). Harmful bacteria, for example, may cause disease through infection of their host or by the release of powerful toxins. Viruses, inert by themselves, have the ability to invade the cells of other life-forms. As those cells duplicate, so does the virus. While one's ability to ward off disease is usually strong, there are instances where the microbes overwhelm the body and produce illness. In an effort to protect against many infectious diseases, we rely on vaccines with the intent of conferring protection and immunity.

Vaccines have been a vehicle for disease prevention and eradication for hundreds of years. The development and widespread distribution of safe, effective, and affordable vaccines has done more for disease prevention over time than nearly any other medical or public health intervention. Of the ten greatest public health achievements over time, certainly immunization against disease ranks at or near the top of the list.[2] Millions of lives have been saved because of the widespread use of vaccines to prevent or eradicate diseases such as measles, diphtheria, pertussis, tetanus, polio, and of course smallpox. The eradication of smallpox worldwide is undoubtedly one of the most spectacular public health initiatives of all time.

Vaccination not only protects an individual from disease, but it also has the dual role of protecting the community at large from disease outbreaks. For disease to spread there must be a pool of susceptible people in whom the bacteria or virus can grow. Ironically, those who elect not to vaccinate themselves or their children are actually benefiting from those who are vaccinated. This concept is referred to as "herd immunity." When a disease spreads from one human to another, it requires both an infected person to spread it and a susceptible person to catch it. Herd immunity works by decreasing the number of susceptible individuals, and when this number drops low enough, the disease will disappear from the community because there are not enough people to continue the catch-and-infect cycle. The greater the proportion of vaccinated individuals, the more rapidly the disease will disappear. Once-common diseases such as pertussis, polio, smallpox, and measles have all but disappeared thanks to the large numbers of individuals who are vaccinated against these diseases. Periodically, however, there have been mini-outbreaks of disease for which there are vaccinations. For example, there continue to be outbreaks of measles (a particularly contagious, potentially serious disease) in the United States as well as around the world, primarily as a result of a pool of unvaccinated children. Those who are not vaccinated are at high risk of contracting this disease.[3]

Because microbes know no foreign boundary, diseases in one part of the world can quickly and easily spread to other parts of the globe. As such, a unified global vaccination policy is needed; how to achieve such a noble and important goal, however, is often not easily accomplished. Economics, politics, and social constraints can and do play important roles in disease-eradication programs. The success of immunization policies depends on, and is linked with, interrelated factors including vaccine safety (quality control and monitoring); adequate vaccine supply (to avoid vaccine shortages), effective delivery systems to ensure that the vaccines get to those in need (more of an issue in the developing world), financial incentives and legal protection for the vaccine manufacturers, and educational efforts to inform the public about the benefits and risks of vaccinations. Indeed, perhaps most of all, there is a need to focus on the public's fears about the safety of vaccination and their willingness to be immunized.

In addition to the scientific challenges to vaccine development, social, ethical, economic, legal, and political issues individually and collectively have served to curtail and in some cases to derail efforts to immunize populations. Vociferous antivaccination movements frequently clashed with the government's authority to immunize for the "common good." Historically, antivaccinationists have protested against what they consider the intrusion of their privacy and bodily integrity. One of the potent symbols of the early antivaccine movement was the limp "raggedy Ann" doll, which was created in 1915 by a man whose daughter died shortly after being vaccinated at school without parental consent. The medical authorities blamed a heart defect, but the parents blamed their child's death on the shot. Since that time, there have been reports of deep-seated public fears of vaccinations, as well as protests against compulsory vaccination laws.

The issue of vaccine safety periodically makes front-page news, usually after an unfortunate event in which someone or many individuals were harmed in some way allegedly as a result of being vaccinated. Proponents of vaccination would be the last to say that vaccination is risk free, but they would be the first to argue that the small risks outweigh the dangers of not being vaccinated. To lose ground to the tremendous achievements realized by vaccines because of the public's mistrust could be potentially serious. Are the antivaccinationists off-base or are their concerns valid? How should the public health and medical communities respond? What role should government have to legally enforce vaccination policy? This chapter focuses on the history of vaccines and immunization and the new challenges that must be addressed to ensure against resurgence in vaccine-preventable diseases locally, nationally, and globally.

## WHAT ARE VACCINES AND HOW DO THEY WORK?

The doctrine holding that infectious diseases are caused by the activity of microorganisms within the body is referred to as the germ theory of disease, also called the pathogenic theory of medicine, which states that microorganisms are the cause of many diseases. Although highly controversial when first proposed in the nineteenth century, it is now a cornerstone of modern medicine and clinical microbiology. Put simply, disease-causing organisms, be they viruses, microbes, or bacteria, attack the body and produce illness. The immune system, if working correctly, prevents illness by destroying disease-causing microorganisms that threaten the body.

Vaccines, from the Latin word "vacca," or cow, trigger one's immune system's infection-fighting ability and memory without exposure to the actual disease-producing germs. Instead, the person is injected with a dead or much weakened (and not dangerous) version of the pathogen. Vaccines stimulate the body's immune system by triggering an immune response; the immune system goes into high gear to destroy the invader. The immunity one develops following vaccination is similar to the immunity acquired from natural infection. For some diseases, several doses of a vaccine (a booster) may be needed for a full immune response. For others, one shot is sufficient.

One's body can become immune to bacteria or viruses by either developing a natural immunity to the disease or by vaccine-induced immunity. *Natural immunity* develops after one has been exposed to an organism, and one's immune system develops a defense (from antibodies and memory cells) to prevent one from getting sick again from that particular type of virus or bacterium. *Vaccine-induced immunity* results after one receives a vaccine, which makes the body think that it is being invaded by a specific organism and the immune system reacts by destroying the "invader" and preventing it from infecting the person again. The immunity one develops following vaccination is similar to the immunity acquired from natural infection. The goal is the same: to stimulate an immune response without causing disease.

Briefly, the human immune system works because antigens (proteins from the foreign microorganism) stimulate an immune response leading to the synthesis of antibodies (proteins that attack and destroy viral or bacterial particles). "Memory cells" are produced in an immune response, and these cells remain in the bloodstream ready to mount a quick protective immune response against subsequent infections with the particular disease-causing agent.[4] If the infection was to occur again, the memory cells would respond to inactivate the disease-causing agents, and the individual would not likely become sick.

Vaccines have traditionally been classified into three broad categories: live attenuated, whole-killed, and subunit vaccines.

- Live weakened vaccines use live viruses that have been weakened (attenuated). The result is a strong antibody response that establishes lifelong immunity, but live, attenuated vaccines carry the greatest risk because they can mutate back to the virulent form at any time. Because the pathogen is alive, it has the potential to multiply within the human body. Examples include vaccines for measles, mumps, and rubella and chickenpox.
- Inactivated vaccines use killed or inactivated bacteria or viruses. Examples included the typhoid vaccine and the Salk poliomyelitis vaccine. Toxoid vaccines use bacterial toxins that have been rendered harmless to provide immunity to the specific toxin. Examples included diphtheria and tetanus vaccines.
- Acellular and subunit vaccines are made by using only part of the virus or bacteria. Advances in biotechnology and genetic engineering techniques have made it possible to produce subunit vaccines in which genes that code for appropriate subunits from the genome of the infectious agent are isolated and placed into bacteria or yeast host cells, which then produce large quantities of subunit molecules by transcribing and translating the inserted foreign DNA. Subunit vaccines cannot cause the disease. Examples include hepatitis B and *Haemophilus influenza* type B vaccines. A booster every few years is often required to continue effectiveness.

## IT ALL STARTED WITH COWPOX

No discussion of vaccines can be considered complete without a discussion of smallpox and Edward Jenner, a country doctor in England who is credited with performing the world's first vaccination in 1796.[5] Jenner observed that milkmaids who had cowpox (a mild disease) rarely developed smallpox (a serious and potentially fatal disease). This observation prompted him to experiment and ultimately devise the first vaccine to protect individuals from this dreaded disease. But, long before Jenner intentionally infected a boy who had recovered from cowpox with smallpox, and long before the causes of this disease were known and understood, many tried to protect the population from this disfiguring and deadly disease.

The Chinese may have begun intentionally infecting themselves with smallpox virus as early as the tenth century, trying to prevent the disease by exposing uninfected individuals to the pus and fluid from a smallpox lesion. The thinking was that the dried pus would confer protection to the individual. This practice, called variolation, was also used hundreds of years later in other parts of the world.[6] Specifically, in the early eighteenth century, Lady Mary Wortley Montagu, the wife of the British ambassador to Constantinople, who as a young girl contracted smallpox and whose brother died of the disease, popularized variolation upon her return to England. Because of Lady Montagu's efforts, the Princess of Wales in 1722 was persuaded to have her two children inoculated against smallpox. Although the physiological effects of variolation varied, ranging from a mild illness to death, its effectiveness was evident. Smallpox mortality and morbidity rates were lower in populations that used variolation than in those who did not.

Across the Atlantic Ocean, smallpox was threatening Boston. Clergyman Cotton Mather and Dr. Zabdiel Boylston in Massachusetts practiced variolation in an attempt to inoculate residents of this city. Although inoculations were illegal in the American colonies, their efforts helped prevent a wide scale smallpox epidemic. They documented that the smallpox case fatality rate was much lower among those inoculated than those not inoculated.[7]

Although Jenner was not the first to experiment with inoculation against smallpox, his efforts, which most certainly would be considered to be unethical by today's standards, are acknowledged to mark the beginning of widespread vaccination. He observed that milkmaids who had cowpox were somehow immune to smallpox. Jenner's experiment on eight-year-old James Phipps spared the boy from developing smallpox, but still Jenner's peers did not readily accept his findings. Rebuffed by the Royal Society of London, Jenner was undeterred and completed more experiments and self-published his findings in 1798. His results were so compelling that thousands of people elected to protect themselves by infecting themselves with cowpox. Though it took several years until Jenner's theories about vaccination were accepted by the professional societies, by 1800, more than 100,000 people had been vaccinated against smallpox worldwide. Vaccination was made compulsory in Bavaria, Denmark, Sweden, and by the mid-nineteenth century, in Great Britain.[8] Massachusetts was the first U.S. state to make vaccination compulsory in 1809.[9]

## MILESTONES IN VACCINE HISTORY

It was almost 100 years after Jenner's seminal work that vaccination moved beyond smallpox. The French chemist, Louis Pasteur, developed what he called a rabies vaccine in 1885, but technically what he produced was a rabies

antitoxin that functioned as a postinfection antidote.[10] By the twentieth
century, advances in the science of virology, bacteriology, and immunology
led to a better understanding of how the human body defends itself against
invading microorganisms. Development of viral vaccines and bacteria-based
vaccines flourished; the development of vaccines against more than twenty
diseases has impacted disease morbidity and mortality. Since 1980, more than
fifteen new or improved vaccines have been approved as a result of advances
in molecular biology and genetics, which led to new and improved subunit
vaccines that promise to offer increased safety and efficacy. (See Table 11.1
for highlights in vaccine development and Table 11.2 for a listing of currently
recommended childhood vaccinations.)

Vaccines have been developed for scores of diseases. Listed herein are just
some of the highlights in history of vaccine development.

### Smallpox

The eradication of smallpox is probably the world's greatest success story.
For thousands of years, epidemics swept across continents, decimating populations and at times changing the course of history. The Crusaders brought

**Table 11.1**
**Highlights in vaccine development**

| | |
|------|--------------------------------------------------------------------------|
| 1905 | U.S. Supreme Court upholds state law mandating smallpox vaccination. |
| 1944 | Pertussis vaccine recommended for universal use in infants. |
| 1947 | DPT (trivalent diphtheria/pertussis/tetanus) recommended for routine use. |
| 1955 | Salk inactivated polio vaccine licensed. |
| 1961 | Sabin oral, live-virus polio vaccine licensed. |
| 1963 | Measles vaccine licensed. |
| 1971 | MMR (trivalent measles/mumps/rubella) licensed. |
| 1972 | United States ended routine use of smallpox vaccine. |
| 1977 | Smallpox eradicated worldwide. |
| 1986 | Vaccine Injury Compensation Act passed. |
| | Recombinant Hepatitis B vaccine licensed (recommended for all newborns and children in 1991). |
| 1988 | Vaccine Injury Compensation Program funded. |
| 1999/ 2000 | Joint statement by the U.S. Public Health Service, the American Associa-tion of Family Practitioners, the American Association of Pediatrics urged manufacturers to remove the preservative thimerosal as soon as possible from vaccines routinely recommended for infants. |

*Source:* National Vaccine Information Center. www.909shots.com/timeline.html.

**Table 11.2**
**Recommended Vaccinations**

| | |
|---|---|
| By age 6 | Measles, mumps, rubella, polio, chicken pox, DPT (diphtheria, tetanus, pertussis), Hib (meningitis), PCV (pneumonia), rotavirus (diarrhea), hepatitis A and B, flu (annually). |
| By age 18 | Meningococcus, cervical cancer (girls only; an HPV vaccine for boys is being developed). |
| Ages 18–65 | Flu (annually), tetanus and diphtheria (every 10 years), measles, mumps, rubella, chicken pox (for those not previously infected), pneumococcal pneumonia flu (annually by age 65). |

*Source:* Centers for Disease Control and Prevention. January 2007.
*Note:* The CDC has updated its recommended list of vaccines several times over the past fifteen years. Each state, rather than the CDC, decides which vaccines to make compulsory for entry into school.

smallpox back with them from the Holy Land. The Conquistadors carried it to the New World. The Incan and Aztec empires were destroyed by this disease. In the American colonies, smallpox helped decimate the indigenous peoples, including Pocahontas who died of smallpox in 1617 after visiting London. Rich and poor, famous and unknown, smallpox did not discriminate. Queen Mary II of England, Emperor Joseph I of Austria, King Luis I of Spain, Tsar Peter II of Russia, and King Louis XV of France are a few of the heads of state who died from smallpox. The disease, for which no effective treatment was ever developed, killed as many as 30% of those infected. Between 65%–80% of survivors were marked with deep-pitted scars (pockmarks), most prominent on the face. George Washington, for example, survived a bout with smallpox but was severely scarred.

By the mid-twentieth century, 150 years after the introduction of vaccination, an estimated 50 million cases of smallpox occurred in the world each year, a figure that dropped to around 10–15 million by 1967 because of successful vaccination efforts. In 1967, when the World Health Organization (WHO) launched an intensified plan to eradicate smallpox from the earth, the "ancient scourge" threatened 60% of the world's population, killed every fourth victim, scarred or blinded most survivors, and eluded any form of treatment.[11] A massive, worldwide outbreak search and vaccination program was initiated and through the success of this global eradication campaign, smallpox was finally limited to the horn of Africa and then to a single last natural case, which occurred in Somalia in 1977, although a fatal laboratory-acquired case occurred in the United Kingdom in 1978. The global eradication of smallpox was certified by a commission of eminent scientists in December 1979, based on intense verification activities in countries, and subsequently was endorsed by the WHO in 1980. Three known repositories of the virus were left: one in Birmingham, England, which was later destroyed after an accidental escape from containment caused many deaths, and two still remaining for possible anti-bioweaponry (stored under extremely strict conditions at the Centers for Disease Control and Prevention in Atlanta, Georgia, and at the State Research Center of Virology and Biotechnology in Koltsovo, Russia).

## Pertussis and Diphtheria

Although the causative agent of pertussis (whooping cough) was isolated in 1907, it was not until the late 1920s that the first whole-killed pertussis vaccine was introduced.[12] Pertussis, particularly serious among infants, is a contagious respiratory disease caused by the *B. pertussis* bacterium and spread by coughing or sneezing. Toxins produced by *B. pertussis* can cause high fever, convulsions, brain damage, and death.

Diphtheria, also caused by a bacterium, is a very contagious and potentially life-threatening infection that usually attacks the throat and nose. In more serious cases, it can attack the nerves and heart. Although he survived smallpox, George Washington may have died of diphtheria. In the mid-1930s, a vaccine against pertussis and diphtheria was developed, and was later modified in 1947 to include tetanus (DPT vaccine). Today, the DPT shot is among the first that an infant receives after birth. A child needs five DPT shots, given at specified intervals, to ensure complete protection.

The DPT booster vaccine was put into widespread use in the late 1950s; however, serious adverse reactions including convulsions, brain damage, and even death were noted in a tiny percentage of children who were vaccinated. In particular, the pertussis component of the DPT vaccine was identified as causing problems in some children. As a result, children with a history of convulsions or neurological disease were strongly advised not to be vaccinated.[13–15] Although serious acute neurologic illness was a rare event, the Institute of Medicine (IOM) was mandated by Congress to study the issue. In 1991, the IOM issued its report and concluded that the evidence was insufficient to indicate a causal relation between DPT and neurologic damage.[16] The National Childhood Encephalopathy Study (NCES) also found that children who experienced rare but serious acute neurologic disorders within seven days of receiving DPT were no more or less likely to experience documented chronic nervous system dysfunction or to have died within ten years of the acute disorder than children who had not received DPT within seven days prior to the onset of the disorder. In sum, there were no special characteristics associated with acute or chronic nervous system illnesses linked to DPT exposure.[17] But, the public's trust was shaken.

## Polio

Probably no disease created as much fear as polio, which primarily affected children. Paralysis and death were the major hazards of this disease. Probably the most famous polio victim in the United States, perhaps even in the world, was President Franklin D. Roosevelt, who hid the extent of his disability from the public throughout his presidency. Polio was one of the most dreaded child-hood diseases of the twentieth century. The first clinical description of polio dates to 1789 when a British physician provided the first description of the disease (debility of the lower extremities). The first known large epidemic occurred in 1916, killing 6,000 people and leaving 27,000 more paralyzed.[18] In retrospect, isolation and quarantine were not effective means of controlling the disease. A race to develop an effective polio vaccine began in the 1930s, and unfortunately early clinical trials failed in that many individuals ended up infected with polio. Clearly, this was not the intent of the vaccine developers. Widespread epidemics of polio were documented after World War II, with an average of more than 20,000 cases a year occurring between 1945 and 1949. In 1952, there were 58,000 cases of polio in the United States, the most ever counted. By the mid-twentieth century, it may not be an exaggeration to say that polio hysteria fueled fear across the country.

The difficulty in developing a polio vaccine stemmed from the fact that this disease is caused by three strains of virus. Understanding the polioviruses took decades, with much of the research funded by the March of Dimes Foundation, a grassroots organization founded with the help of President Roosevelt. In the late 1940s, Dr. Jonas Salk began to use the newly developed tissue cultures method of cultivating and working with the poliovirus. The first safe and effective vaccine, the Salk injected vaccine, used killed poliovirus. During the 1950s, massive field trials of the Salk vaccine, unprecedented in medical history, were conducted and led to a nationwide mass immunization campaign promoted by the March of Dimes. This effort led to a significant drop in the number of new cases of polio in the United States, and in 1955, the inactivated polio vaccine was licensed for use in the United States. While the vaccine helped stop polio in its tracks, there were problems with the vaccine relating to the incomplete inactivation of some virus particles. This was soon corrected.

During this time, Dr. Albert Sabin, a bitter rival of Salk, also was working on a polio vaccine. His vaccine used live, attenuated (weakened) virus rather than killed poliovirus. Whereas the Salk vaccine required injections, the Sabin vaccine was oral. Field trials of this vaccine proved the Sabin oral vaccine to be effective; the oral, live-virus polio vaccine was licensed in 1961. Because live vaccine contains a weakened type of poliovirus that could in theory mutate into more virulent forms (albeit exceedingly rare, but not unheard of), it is not given to people with impaired immune systems. The oral vaccine was superior in terms of ease of administration, and it also provided longer-lasting immunity. Both vaccines have advantages and disadvantages with regard to safety and cost, and both are used throughout the world.

The discovery and use of the polio vaccines nearly eliminated polio in the United States, and in 1994, this disease was declared eradicated in all of the Americas. While both the Salk and the Sabin vaccines proved to be highly effective in preventing the disease, those who had been paralyzed by polio, estimated to be in the hundred of thousands, unfortunately did not benefit from these milestones in polio vaccine development.

## Measles, Mumps, and Rubella

As late as the 1950s, and before a vaccine was developed, parents were encouraged to expose their children to diseases like measles, mumps, and chicken pox to develop immunity. With the marketing of an effective vaccine to protect people from these diseases, such thinking was rendered moot. Building on the momentum of success achieved with the oral polio vaccine, a number of live attenuated vaccines were being developed. The most significant of these at the time was the measles-mumps-rubella (MMR) vaccine.

For hundreds of years, measles was so ubiquitous it was thought to be a natural episode of childhood. It was not until the fourteenth century that the word "measles" was used, stemming from the word "miser," which was used to refer to the wretchedness of lepers.[19] Prior to the development of an effective vaccine, measles was one of the most common childhood diseases in America. Characterized by fever and a rash, measles is a serious disease that is highly contagious and can lead to death; but recovery confers a lifelong immunity. Interestingly, women who have been vaccinated but who never had the disease do not have natural maternal measles antibodies to pass on to their babies, which mean that most babies born in America are vulnerable to getting this disease.

Mumps, a viral disease, also used to be very common in childhood. Discovery of the mumps virus in 1934 helped researchers gain a better understanding of the symptoms and how this disease is transmitted. Characterized by fever, headache, and inflammation of the salivary glands (making the cheeks swell producing the signature sign of the disease), this disease rarely leads to death. Recovery confers lifelong immunity.

Rubella (German measles) is usually a mild childhood disease characterized by a pink rash. While similar to measles, the rubella virus is comparatively benign and less infectious. Recovery usually confers lifelong immunity although repeat cases can occur, albeit rarely. Should a pregnant woman get rubella in the first trimester of pregnancy, there is a greater chance of giving birth to a baby with birth defects.

While a measles vaccine was licensed in 1963, and a rubella vaccine was licensed in 1969, the trivalent MMR vaccine was licensed in 1971. Protection is estimated to last for up to eleven years. Despite the availability of the vaccine, however, around 1 million children, predominantly in resource-poor countries, die every year from measles. Even in the United States, outbreaks occur. For example, a measles outbreak in the 1980s and early 1990s showed that there were a significant number of vaccine failures in older children, teenagers, and adults, especially among those who had been vaccinated before fifteen months of age. As such, the government recommended that a second MMR booster be given either before a child enters kindergarten or before entering junior high school. Almost all who get the vaccine have no serious adverse reactions from it.

As is often the case, the risks of the vaccine are usually smaller than the risks from the diseases. However, in the mid-1990s, reports of an association between autism and the MMR vaccine were published. There was speculation that the MMR vaccination could cause autism in some children. This finding alarmed both the lay public and the scientific community. Parents refused to have their children immunized, and the IOM was asked to investigate this link. More on this later.

## Influenza ("Flu")

During World War I, the number of American killed by influenza (44,000) almost was equal to the number killed in battle (50,000). As the nation entered World War II, the military decided to make influenza vaccination mandatory. Influenza is a contagious disease spread by person-to-person contact and caused by the influenza virus. Peak flu season occurs usually from late December through March. There are three basic flu germs, variants of which are popularly designated according to where they first strike; that is, Hong Kong B, Bangkok A, and so forth. It's important to remember that influenza viruses are constantly changing, so an antibody made against one strain will become less effective against new strains as influenza strains evolve over time. In addition, there are different types of influenza viruses circulating and different variants within virus types, and the same type of flu virus does not necessarily circulate each year. For instance, during the 2005–06 flu season, influenza A (H3N2) viruses predominated; however, infection with influenza A (H3N2) virus would not provide protection against influenza B or influenza A (H1N1) viruses. The viruses that cause flu are prone to mutation, making the manufacture of vaccines an annual guessing game of sorts. If a new mutation pops up anywhere in the world, resulting from a major change (antigenic "shift"), it will quickly spread, leaving most people unprotected.

Historically, influenza epidemics have cased havoc. Charlemagne's army may have been decimated by the flu during an epidemic in 876. The great influenza pandemic of 1918–19, the twentieth century's worst epidemic, killed millions of people. A flu shot can help prevent one from getting sick, but even with the flu vaccine available, each year millions of people get sick, and some tens of thousands die from the flu. When complicated by pneumonia, it is one of the ten most common causes of death in the United States. Most people who get a flu shot have no serious problem from the vaccination. Those over age sixty are recommended to get a flu shot every year.

## Hepatitis

Hippocrates was the first to note epidemics of jaundice, a telltale characteristic of hepatitis. Today we know that hepatitis is a gastroenterological disease featuring inflammation of the liver. Most cases of acute hepatitis are due to viral infections. There are many types of hepatitis, and the disease can be contracted in a few different ways. *Hepatitis A* is transmitted by the orofecal route and is contracted through contaminated food or water. This form of hepatitis does not lead to chronic or life long disease and just about everyone who gets hepatitis A has a full recovery.

*Hepatitis B* can be contracted from blood, semen, and saliva (making it one of the venereal diseases) and also from tattoos. Hepatitis B can be a serious infection that can cause liver damage; some individuals are not able to get rid of the virus, which makes the infection chronic. Before routine testing of the blood supply, thousands of deaths occurred each year from post-transfusion hepatitis B. Fortunately, this is no longer a risk.

*Hepatitis C* is spread the same way as hepatitis B through an infected person's blood and other body fluids as well, as from injection drug use. Hepatitis C is a chronic infection and often causes liver damage. *Hepatitis D* can only thrive is cells also infected with hepatitis B and is not very common. It can be spread through infected blood, dirty needles, and from unprotected sex with a person infected with hepatitis virus. *Hepatitis E* can be contracted from host to host via fecal–oral contact and contamination of water. This type of hepatitis does not occur often in the United States and does not confer long-term damage to the liver. In 1991, a recombinant hepatitis B vaccine was recommended for all newborn infants and children. There is no vaccine for hepatitis C, D, or E.

## Human Papillomavirus (HPV)

HPVs are the most common sexually transmitted infections in the United States. Sexually transmitted HPVs, common in adults and sexually active adolescents, more often than not are harmless and come and go without causing any symptoms. However, there is a subset of nineteen "high risk" HPV types that can lead to the development of cervical cancer and genital warts. Whereas genital warts can cause discomfort and psychosocial trauma, cervical cancer, if not detected in the early stages, can be deadly. Therefore, a vaccine that would protect against these diseases, especially cervical cancer, would be very beneficial indeed. In 2006, the FDA approved the first preventive HPV vaccine marketed by Merck and Co. under the trade name Gardasil. Gardasil, a recombinant vaccine (contains no live virus), is a preventive rather than a therapeutic vaccine and is recommended for women who are between nine and 25 years old who do not have HPV. The vaccine will not protect a woman if she has been infected with HPV types prior to the vaccination, indicating the importance of getting immunized before potential exposure to the virus (before initiation of sexual activity). A series of three shots over a six-month period was shown to offer 100% protection against the development of cervical pre-cancers and genital warts caused by the HPV types in the vaccine. The protective effects of the vaccine are expected to last a minimum of four and a half years after the initial vaccination.

The vaccine represents a significant advance in the protection of women's health. There are, however, a couple of drawbacks to the vaccine that have sparked debate. First, the vaccine is expensive. Second, the vaccine offers no protection against other specific types of HPV that can also cause cervical cancer (there are more than 120 known HPV types, and 27 are known to be transmitted through sexual contact). The vaccine targets two of the most common high-risk HPVs, type 16 and 18, which cause 70% of all cervical cancers, and HPV types 6 and 11, which cause about 90% of all cases of genital warts. Third, it is unknown whether the vaccine's protection against HPV-16, in particular, is long-lasting. Fourth, since the vaccine works only against specific kinds of HPV, regular Pap tests should still be performed. And, fifth, the vaccine is targeted only to females, leaving the males to serve as an asymptomatic reservoir for the virus.

Perhaps the most contentious issue of HPV vaccination is the recommendation to vaccinate young girls. Social conservative religious groups have publicly opposed the concept of making HPV vaccination mandatory for pre-adolescent girls because they fear that this might send a subtle message that sexual intercourse is okay, thus detracting from their abstinence-based position. Other critics question *mandating* the vaccine for young girls. Many parents are extremely uncomfortable at the notion of vaccinating their young daughters against a sexually transmitted disease. But the reality is that the vaccine will not work after a woman has been infected, so the thinking is that it is preferable to have the young girl vaccinated before she becomes sexually active. Not surprisingly, there is heated debate as to whether the vaccinations should be required or recommended. Proponents argue that the objections are not strong enough to forgo the protection against a potentially dangerous disease.

Texas is the first state to require vaccinating girls ages 11 and 12. The governor, a conservative Republican, has endorsed this position but has left the door open for parents to "opt out" by petitioning for an exemption for reasons of conscience or religious beliefs. Whether other states will follow Texas' lead remains to be seen. What is clear is that this new vaccine has been shown to have the ability to protect females from a serious disease.

## THE IMPORTANCE OF VACCINATION AND RESISTANCE TO IT

The marketing of Gardasil and similar prototypes in the pipeline illustrates that pharmaceutical companies and biotech companies are engaged in vaccine research. With the advancement of molecular biology and genetics, vaccine development continues to grow at an exciting rate. New and improved subunit vaccines that promise to offer increased safety and high efficacy are being studied. Additionally, novel strategies for vaccine delivery, especially the elimination of needles, as well as the combination of multiple vaccine components to different pathogens into a single vaccine delivery (of note, the MMR and the

DPT vaccines) hold great promise. Yet, there has been, and continues to be, resistance to immunization among some groups of individuals. Indeed, vaccine development has had its share of political drama and controversy over time.

In England, Jenner's experiments were so compelling that lawmakers moved to make vaccination compulsory; in 1853, a law was passed requiring vaccination for smallpox for all infants within the first year of life. Parents who did not vaccinate their children were subject to fine and imprisonment. Immediately, an Anti-Vaccination League was formed in London, and members of this league included all socioeconomic classes.

Liberal intellectuals argued that the law violated individual liberty, and religious leaders proclaimed that injecting animal disease into children was "un-Christian."[20] Those in the working class felt that vaccination threatened the control of their own and their children's bodies.[21] Fear and ignorance prevailed, as many believed that vaccination could spread disease and cause death. In retrospect, perhaps these individuals were not so off base, as the unhygienic methods prevalent at the time could and did indeed spread disease from one person to the next.

Many children were not vaccinated, which prompted new legislation to toughen enforcement. The 1871 Vaccination Act required each district to appoint vaccination officers (nonmedical personnel) who were paid to find noncompliers and impose fines.[22] Almost 200 antivaccination groups were active during the 1880s in England, and numerous demonstrations were held in protest of the law.[23] At one demonstration, an effigy of Edward Jenner was hanged and then decapitated!

The antivaccination movement prompted Parliament to create a Royal Commission to investigate the utility and safety of smallpox vaccine. In 1896, the Commission concluded that vaccination did indeed protect against smallpox, but recommended relaxing penalties against resistors.[24] The Vaccination Act of 1898 included a conscience clause that permitted citizens who did not believe in vaccination to obtain an exemption certificate for their children. This act actually introduced the idea of "conscientious objector" into English law.[25]

Following the English experience, numerous states in the United States drafted vaccination laws. In response, an antivaccination movement was born in America.[26] The American antivaccination movement focused on the concept of "inalienable rights," and its proponents argued that vaccination opposed the laws of nature and religious laws.[27] Aggressive campaigns to repeal vaccination requirements were held in numerous states. Some antivaccination activists went so far as to argue that smallpox was not contagious, and a few tried to prove this by intentionally exposing themselves to the disease, usually with disastrous results. Taking a lead role in the antivaccination movement were the patent medicine manufacturers, who feared (probably correctly) that vaccination laws would ruin their business.

By 1905, eleven states had passed laws requiring vaccination, but three-quarters of these states did not have any legal penalties for those who chose not to comply.[28] In a challenge to the constitutionality of the Massachusetts law requiring vaccination, the Supreme Court ruled in 1905 in a landmark case, *Jacobson v. Massachusetts*, that the need to protect the public health through compulsory smallpox vaccination outweighed the individual's right to privacy.[29] The Court affirmed the state's right to require vaccination as part of its police powers and asserted that within reasonable limits, individual interests were superseded by the health of the public. This decision laid the groundwork for subsequent public health law in the United States.[30] Further, in 1922, the Supreme Court upheld the compulsory school entry vaccination laws.[31] Yet, whenever a new vaccine was introduced, including diphtheria and typhoid fever in the 1920s, polio in the 1950s, and measles, rubella, pertussis, and hepatitis in the later part of the twentieth century, groups opposed to vaccination would appear on the scene.

## VACCINATION AND SCHOOL POLICY

The American Academy of Pediatrics issued their first immunization guidelines in the 1930s. But, the public health initiative to create school laws requiring vaccination began in the 1960s and 1970s, after the polio epidemic of the 1950s. By 1963, twenty states required immunization as a requirement for school entrance, and this number grew to twenty-nine by 1970.[32] Many of these laws were created and enforced to protect against measles, in particular. Data showed that states with school immunization laws had 40%–51% lower rates of measles than states without such laws.[33,34] Such data were compelling and provided the impetus for the remaining states to enact and enforce school immunization laws. As these laws are state-based, variations exist in requirements and enforcement. By 2006, all states allowed medical exemptions, forty-eight had a provision for religious exemptions, and nineteen permitted "personal belief" exemptions.[35] "Personal belief" exemptions refer to religious, philosophical, and any other undetermined exemptions that are not medical. Interestingly, a study looking into the effect of such exemptions on disease outbreaks found that states with "personal belief" exemptions had a 27% higher rate of new pertussis cases than states without such an exemption.[36] Moreover, enforcement of school vaccination laws varied significantly at the local school level. Schools with simplified or inexplicit exemption claim procedures, as well as schools allowing philosophical exemptions, had increased exemption rates and higher risk of disease outbreaks.

## PROTESTING VACCINES: FACT OR MYTH

Antivaccination movements often can have a significant effect on public health, primarily as a result of outbreaks of vaccine-preventable diseases. But, are the fears and concerns of the antivaccination movement unwarranted? What is the trade-off between benefit and risk? While nineteenth- and early

twentieth-century fears of vaccination might have been based on anecdotal hor-
ror stories, vaccine safety is a real and constant concern. New vaccines and
vaccine combinations that provide a wider array of protection from diseases
often require more injections, which, in rare cases, may lead to serious reactions. As with other pharmaceutical products, vaccines can produce side effects
ranging from local injection-site soreness or redness to low-grade fevers, to
more serious adverse events. Therefore, safety concerns are not entirely off
base. Public health experts believe that the system of routine childhood immunizations rests on a tenuous foundation of public support. Primarily because
the success of immunization programs depends on parents' beliefs that vaccinating their children is safer than not doing so, it is imperative that parents and
the public understand the risks as well as the benefits of vaccination.

Yet, all it takes is the hint of vaccine-safety controversy to scare off people
from getting vaccinated. For example, in 1976, there was a scare that the swine
influenza vaccine was associated with a severe paralytic illness called Guillain-
Barré Syndrome (GBS). During the 1976–77 swine influenza vaccination
campaign, for example, 1,300 cases of GBS were reported to the CDC.[37]
According to the CDC's vaccine information sheet on the influenza vaccine, if
there is a risk of GBS from this influenza vaccine, it is estimated at one or two
cases per million persons vaccinated, much less than the risk of severe influenza. Nevertheless, at that time, fear of developing GBS after a flu shot heightened distrust of getting an influenza vaccination. It is important to stress that
most people who get the influenza vaccine have no serious problem from it.

Also in the 1970s, when there was a suggested connection between the DPT
vaccine and neurological damage in children, acceptance of this vaccine plum-
meted resulting in a widespread resurgence of pertussis, especially in Great
Britain where parents refused to have their children immunized.[38] Many
parents who chose not to vaccinate their children doubted the reliability of vaccination information from authorities, believing that doctors overestimate protection and underestimate dangers of vaccines.[39] Further, vaccines have been
so effective that many parents, thankfully, have never seen cases of diseases
against which vaccines protect, which in a sense diminishes the vaccine's perceived value and creates apathy.[40] A survey showed that 25% of those polled
felt that children receive more vaccines than needed.[41] Between 1990 and
2000, for example, vaccines against four diseases (*Haemophilus influenza* type
B, hepatitis B, chicken pox, and pneumococcal disease), entailing ten to twelve
injections, were added to the immunization schedule. Parents felt that children
were becoming "pediatric pin cushions."[42]

The antivaccination movement, both in the United States and abroad, has
been facilitated by the Internet, a fertile breeding ground for dissemination of
information, both correct and incorrect. Several studies have evaluated the
information posted on the Internet, and the results are troubling. One study
found that almost 43% of online sites about the MMR vaccine were negative
and contained inaccurate and unbalanced information.[43] The most frequently

cited incorrect information was that vaccines cause other illnesses such as neu-rologic disorders, multiple sclerosis, autism, asthma, and sudden infant death syndrome (SIDS). Other common bits of misinformation were that vaccines contain potentially large amounts of contaminants and mercury.[44]

The media, perhaps unintentionally, also fuels antivaccination sentiments. The power of the media to influence vaccination policy is illustrated by the impact of a British television documentary that aired in 1974 showing children allegedly harmed by vaccines. In the United States, too, a 1982 television spe-cial on the DPT vaccine included interviews with families alleging that their children were brain damaged after being vaccinated. By insinuating a cover-up, the media played into the fears of the antivaccination movement. Though heavily criticized by physicians and scientists, the show won an Emmy!

More recently, in 1998, British scientists, led by Andrew Wakefield, pub-lished an article in *Lancet* suggesting a connection between the MMR vaccine and autism.[45] Before the study (which was based on only twelve cases) could be adequately evaluated by the scientific community, the lay press in both the United Kingdom and the United States picked up on the article. The authors of the article eventually retracted the assertion of a link between the MMR vac-cine and autism, but the public's confidence in the MMR vaccine was certainly shaken. The *Lancet* article was not the first to raise concerns about the MMR vaccine as earlier media reports of litigation by parents who believed that the vaccine had precipitated autism in their previously healthy infants. Immuniza-tion rates for MMR fell despite the British and American governments warning parents not to reject MMR vaccinations. Even when the media reported results of new studies that rejected the link between MMR and autism, the public was still skeptical. An editorial in the *British Medical Journal* stated:

"The media excitement and public concern after a Lancet report linking MMR with autism kindles a sense of déjà vu. It is highly reminiscent of similar scares over pertus-sis in the 1970s, which resulted in much suffering and many deaths, both in Britain and internationally."[46]

For reasons that are not entirely clear, the rates of MMR vaccination dropped significantly in Britain but remained virtually unchanged in the United States. One explanation may relate to the fact that immunizations are voluntary in Great Britain and compulsory in the United States. Also, British physicians were more divided over the alleged risks while physicians in the United States were more unified in their support for the vaccine. Perhaps the press coverage was more inflammatory in the United Kingdom than in the United States. In any event, in the United States, the IOM studied the evidence in two separate reports and conclusively rejected the putative causal relationship between vac-cines and autism spectrum disorders.[47,48]

Another controversy that engaged the antivaccination movement was the use of thimerosal, a mercury-containing organic compound, as a preservative to extend the shelf life of some vaccines. It was suggested that thimerosal in childhood vaccines could contribute to, or cause, a range of neurodevelopmental disorders in children, including attention-deficit/hyperactivity disorder (ADHD). The critics argued that the ethylmercury-based preservative could cause serious side effects when administered to young children who have relatively undeveloped immune and neurological systems. The situation escalated to the point where over 4,000 lawsuits were filed by parents and guardians of children who they allege were affected by thimerosal, despite the lack of epidemiological evidence showing a statistical association between thimerosal and any neurological disorder. A hearing is expected in June 2007.

These concerns provided the impetus for the passage of the Food and Drug Administration (FDA) Modernization Act of 1997, which called for a review and risk assessment of mercury-containing food and drugs. The FDA's Center for Biologics Evaluation and Research (CBER) investigated the issue and found that some children could have exceeded the federal guidelines for single-dose mercury exposure, but the results were inconclusive. A 2004 IOM report on the subject concluded that the evidence did not support a causal relationship between thimerosal-containing vaccines and autism, whereas a Congressional investigation did find evidence that thimerosal posed a risk.[49] Today, the actual amount of thimerosal present in vaccines for children is listed, and usually labeled as "trace" or nil. Currently, adolescent and adult tetanus vaccine and certain influenza vaccines still contain thimerosal.

## ENSURING VACCINE SAFETY AND MONITORING: CHECKS AND BALANCES

Over the next decades, it is estimated that the number of recommended vaccines could exceed fifty-four by the year 2020.[50] The challenge is to minimize the number of injections and minimize the side effects without compromising effectiveness and patient acceptability. However, before the FDA can license any vaccine, it must be assessed for safety and efficacy. Postlicensure studies continue to monitor vaccine safety. Given the problems and adverse effects from vaccines, Congress passed the 1986 National Childhood Vaccine Injury Act, which was spearheaded by parents troubled by a putative link between vaccination and neurological problems. Essentially, the act was designed to reduce the potential financial liability of vaccine makers due to vaccine injury claims and established a no-fault system for litigating claims against vaccine manufacturers. Mounting potential liabilities totaling in the tens of billions of dollars posed financial threats to the pharmaceutical companies who produced vaccines. Vaccine makers indicated that they would cease production if this protection under the law was not enacted. The argument was that public health safety depended on the financial viability of pharmaceutical companies whose ability to produce sufficient supplies of vaccines could be imperiled by civil litigation on behalf of vaccine injury victims.

The act also mandated that all health care providers and manufacturers report certain adverse events following vaccinations to the Vaccine Adverse Event Reporting System (VAERS). Through VAERS, jointly operated by the FDA and the CDC to monitor the safety of licensed vaccines, experts look for patterns and any unusual trends that may raise questions about a vaccine's safety once it is used more widely in the population. The FDA continuously reviews and evaluates individual reports, in addition to monitoring overall reporting patterns. The FDA also monitors reporting trends for individual vaccine lots. Most reports come from health care providers, but anyone can report an unexpected event after vaccination to VAERS. VAERS' role is to generate new hypotheses about the cause of adverse events. For example, in August 1998, a vaccine against the rotavirus became available and infants were immunized. Within a few months, VAERS received reports that fifteen infants developed a rare intestinal condition shortly after receiving the rotavirus vaccine. Although the number was very small in comparison to the number of infants who received the injection, analysis of the VAERS reports and other data suggested that the vaccine might be associated with an increase in the risk of this rare complication and in October 1999, the vaccine was discontinued pending further study.

The Clinical Immunization Safety Assessment Centers (CISA) serve as an additional level of scrutiny of selected patients whose symptoms or diagnoses my represent a new adverse event. The Vaccine Safety Datalink (VSD) provides data from a variety of sources, including immunization records, hospital discharge records, and mortality data.

In 1988, a National Vaccine Injury Compensation Program was created. The program is a federal "no-fault" system designed to compensate those individuals or families of individuals who have been injured by childhood vaccines. A claim may be made for any injury or death thought to be the result of a vaccine covered under the program. The U.S. Department of Health and Human Services, the U.S. Court of Federal Claims, and the U.S. Department of Justice administer the program. But, the program stipulated that all claims against vaccine manufacturers could not be heard in state or federal court, but had to be heard in the U.S. Court of Federal Claims, often referred to as the "vaccine court." Cases are heard without juries, and awards damages are typically far below damage awards rendered in other courts.

In 2006, however, the U.S. Fifth Circuit Court of Appeals ruled that plaintiffs suing three manufacturers of thiomersal could litigate in either state or federal court. This ruling was significant for this, as well as for the fact that the Fifth Circuit Court concluded that thiomersal is not a vaccine but a preservative and the manufacturers cannot share in the protection afforded by the no-fault system of the National Childhood Vaccine Injury Act.

Globally, the WHO has taken steps to ensure vaccine safety by establishing in 1999 the Global Advisory Committee on Vaccine Safety.[51] This committee is charged with advising the WHO on vaccine-related safety issues to enable WHO to respond promptly to issues of vaccine safety. The committee also assesses the implications of vaccine safety worldwide and has weighed in on all of the important vaccine controversies, including MMR and autism, the safety of the mumps vaccine, thiomersal-containing vaccines, and the safety of influenza vaccination for pregnant women.

## NEW CHALLENGES

The successful implementation of mass immunization programs and the subsequent eradication or reduction of smallpox, polio, measles, pertussis, meningococcal meningitis, diphtheria, mumps, rubella, and tetanus are among the most notable public health achievements of the twentieth century. Yet, the path to the eradication of diseases by means of vaccination has not always been smooth. Efforts to develop an effective vaccine against tuberculosis (TB) so far have eluded scientists, although the BCG vaccine is used in many countries, but not in the United States. The parasites responsible for malaria continue to challenge those working on a vaccine for this deadly disease that kills more than 1 million people worldwide each year and infects more than 300 million children a year.[52] Attempts to develop an HIV vaccine to target the retrovirus that causes this disease as well as a vaccine against malaria have so far ended in failure.

Clearly, other challenges remain. Pharmaceutical firms and biotech companies have little incentive to develop vaccines because there is little revenue potential, regulatory barriers, and the exposure to litigation is high should there be adverse events associated with the vaccine. For example, Warner Lambert (now Pfizer) stopped making Fluogen vaccine for influenza in 1998 primarily because of regulatory obstacles and financial loss. Some opine that this led to the flu vaccine shortage in the United States in 2004.[53] Even though the number of vaccines administered has risen dramatically in recent decades, this increase is probably due to government mandates rather than economic incentives. Researchers and policymakers are calling for a different approach to motivate vaccine producers, including offering tax credits or guaranteed purchase, as well as other mechanisms to ensure an adequate vaccine supply and a financial return.[54]

Providing vaccines to the world is a necessary public health challenge that cannot be lost. Despite the monumental successes in vaccine development, the burden of infectious disease remains an important global concern. Fragmented delivery systems and difficulties in tracking and verifying immunization coverage, too, need to be addressed. Minimizing the difficulties in producing, distributing, and administering vaccines and ensuring the safety of the vaccine products should be every government's top priority for disease prevention. As the annual flu outbreaks and anthrax scares remind us, there is a need for new vaccines. It is incumbent upon all governments to ensure that the means and the resources be made available to build on the progress already made to eradicate vaccine-preventable diseases and thereby eliminate unnecessary human suffering worldwide.

# Notes

## CHAPTER 1: ABOUT POLITICS AND SCIENCE

1. Guston, DH. Forget politicizing science. Let's democratize science! *Issues in Science and Technology*. Fall 2004. www.issues.org/21.1/p_guston.html.

2. Pielke, R. Another epidemic of politics? *Science*. 2003;300(5622):1092–1093.

3. Guston, DH. *Between Politics and Science*. Cambridge: Cambridge University Press, 2000.

4. Ibid., p. xv.

5. Silver, HJ. Science and politics: The uneasy relationship. *Open Spaces Quarterly*. 2005;8:1. www.open-spaces.com.

6. Gough, M (ed.). *Politicizing Science: The Alchemy of Policymaking*. Stanford, CA: Hoover Institution Press, 2003.

7. Greenberg, DS. *Science, Money, and Politics: Political Triumph and Ethical Erosion*. Chicago: University of Chicago Press, 2001.

8. Specter, M. The Bush administration's war on the laboratory. *The New Yorker*. March 13, 2006. p. 68.

9. Marshall, E. Hit list at the EPA? *Science*. 1982;219:1303.

10. Hilts, PJ. Ideological tests ruled out in filling U.S. science jobs. *New York Times*. October 30, 1989. p. A1.

11. Lawler, A, and Kaiser, J. Report accuses Bush Administration, again, of "politicizing" science. *Science*. 2004;305:323–325.

12. Blackburn, E. Bioethics and the political distortion of biomedical science. *New Engl J Med*. 2004;350:1379–1380.

13. Keiger, D. Political science. *Johns Hopkins Magazine*. www.jhu.edu/-jhumag/1104web/polisci.html.

14. Union of Concerned Scientists. *Scientific Integrity in Policymaking: An Investigation into the Bush Administration's Misuse of Science*. Cambridge, MA: Union of Concerned Scientists, 2004. www.ucsusa.org.

15. Steinbrook, R. Science, politics, and federal advisory committees. *New Engl J Med*. 2004;350:1454–1461.

16. *Politics and Science in the Bush Administration.* Prepared for Rep. Henry A. Waxman. U.S. House of Representatives. Committee on Government Reform–Minority Staff. Special Investigations Division. August 2003.

17. Stein, R. Internal dissension grows as CDC faces big threats to public health. *Internatl J Health Services.* 2005;35:779–782.

18. Mooney, C. *The Republican War on Science.* New York: Basic Books, 2005.

19. Waxman, HA. *Framing Science: Has Politics Taken Over the Direction of Scientific Research?* Plenary Session of the National Association of Science Writers. February 16, 2005.

20. H.R. 839: Restore Scientific Integrity to Federal Research and Policymaking Act. 109th U.S. Congress. 2005–2006.

## CHAPTER 2: THE POLITICS OF CONTRACEPTION

1. *A History of Birth Control Methods.* www.plannedparenthood.org.

2. Hill, CA. The distinctiveness of sexual motives in relation to sexual desire and desirable partner attributes. *J Sex Research.* 1997;34:139–153.

3. Wilcox, AJ. Timing of sexual intercourse in relation to ovulation. *New Engl J Med.* 1995;333:1517–1521.

4. *A Brief History of Contraception.* www.articles.syl.com/abriefhistory of contraception.html.

5. Asbell, B. *The Pill: A Biography of the Drug That Changed the World.* New York: Random House, 1995.

6. Kennedy, DM. *Birth Control in America: The Career of Margaret Sanger.* New Haven, CT: Yale University Press, 1970.

7. Asbell, B. Op cit.

8. Ibid.

9. Tone, A. *Devices and Desires: A History of Contraceptives in America.* New York: Hill and Wang, 2001.

10. Ibid.

11. Ibid.

12. Connell, EB. Contraception in the prePill era. *Contraception.* 1999;59(1 Suppl): 7S–10S.

13. Bullough, VL, and Bullough, B. *Contraception: A Guide to Birth Control Methods.* Buffalo, NY: Prometheus Press, 1990.

14. Tone, A. Op cit.

15. Perry, S, and Dawson, J. *Nightmare: Women and the Dalkon Shield.* New York: Macmillan, 1985.

16. Hubacher, D. The checkered history and bright future of intrauterine contraception in the United States—viewpoint. *Perspectives on Sexual and Reproductive Health.* 2002;34:98–103.

17. Watkins, ES. *On the Pill: A Social History of Oral Contraception, 1950–1970.* Baltimore: Johns Hopkins University Press, 1998.

18. Djerassi, C. *This Man's Pill: Reflections on the 50th Birthday of the Pill.* New York: Oxford University Press, 2001.

19. Alan Guttmacher Institute. *Teenage Pregnancy: The Problem That Hasn't Gone Away.* New York: Alan Guttmacher Institute, 1981.

20. Boonstra, H, and Nash, E. Minors and the right to consent to health care. *Guttmacher Report on Public Policy*. 2000;3:4–8.

21. Paul, EW, and Pilpel, H. Teenagers and pregnancy: The law in 1979. *Family Plan Persp*. 1979;1:297–302.

22. Finkel, ML. Adolescent sexual behavior and U.S. public policy: Are we meeting the challenge? *Internatl J Adoles Med and Health*. 1985;1:96–105.

23. Green, TL. *Planned Parenthood Funded Study Says Girls Impeded from Use of Sexual Health Services*. Concerned Women for America. 2002. www.cwfa.org.

24. American Medical Association. *Confidential Care for Minors*. 2002. www.ama-assn.org.

25. The Alan Guttmacher Institute. Minors' access to STD services. *State Policies in Brief*. September 10, 2004.

26. The Alan Guttmacher Institute. Minors' access to contraceptive services. *State Policies in Brief*. September 10, 2004.

27. Jones, RK, and Boonstra, H. Confidential reproductive health services for minors: The potential impact of mandated parental involvement for contraception. *Perspectives on Sexual and Reproductive Health*. 2004;36:182–191.

28. Dailard, C. New medical records privacy rule: The interface with teen access to confidential care. *Guttmacher Report on Public Policy*. 2003;6:6–7.

29. The Alan Guttmacher Institute. *Uneven and Unequal: Insurance Coverage and Reproductive Health Services*. New York: Alan Guttmacher Institute, 1994.

30. Sonfield, A, et al. U.S. insurance coverage of contraception and the impact of contraception coverage mandates, 2002. *Perspectives on Sexual and Reproductive Health*. 2004;36:72–80.

31. Western District of Washington. U.S. District Court. *Hennifer Erickson v. Kartell Drug Co*. C.00-12131. June 21, 2001.

32. Mosher, WD, et al. Use of contraception and use of family planning services in the United States: 1982–2002. *Advance Data from Vital and Health Statistics*. Number 350. December 10, 2004.

33. Drazen, J, Greene, MF, Wood, AJJ. The FDA, politics, and plan B. *New Engl J Med*. 2004;350:1561–1562.

34. Ellertson, C. History and efficacy of emergency contraception: Beyond Coca Cola. *Family Plan Persp*. 1996;28:44–48.

35. Grossman, RA, and Grossman, BD. How frequently is emergency contraception prescribed? *Family Plan Persp*. 1994;26:270–271.

36. Kaiser Family Foundation. *Emergency Contraception: Is the Secret Getting Out? National Survey of Americans and Health Care Providers on Emergency Contraception*. www.kff.org/content/archive/1352.

37. *Contraception War*. www.courier-journal.com/apps/pbcs.dll/article?

38. Henshaw, S. Unintended pregnancy in the U.S. *Family Plan Persp*. 1998;30:24–29, 46.

39. Hopkins, J. FDA rejected contraception for political reasons. *BMJ*. 2006;332:624.

40. Hopkins, J. FDA official resigns over emergency contraception decision. *BMJ*. 2005;331:532. And Wood, SF. When politics defeats science. www.washingtonpost.com. March 1, 2006.

41. A sad day for science at the FDA. *New Engl J Med*. (online) 10.1056/NEJM. P058222.

42. Grimes, DA. Emergency contraception: Politics trumps science at the U.S. Food and Drug Administration. *Obstet Gynecol.* 2004;104:220–221.

43. FDA prescription drug products: Certain combined oral contraception for use as postcoital emergency contraception. *Federal Register.* 1997;62137:8609–8612.

44. Grimes, DA, Raymond, EG, and Scott, JB. Emergency contraception over-the-counter: The medical and legal imperative. *Obstet Gynecol.* 2001;98:151–155.

45. Gold, MA, et al. The effects of advance provision of emergency contraception on adolescent women's sexual and contraceptive behavior. *J Pediatr Adoles Gynecol.* 2004;17:87–96.

46. Ackerman, T. Emergency contraception: Science and religion collide. *Annals of Emerg Med.* 2006;47:154–57.

47. Religion at the Drugstore. CBS News Poll. CBS News. November 23, 2004.

48. *U.S. Policy Can Reduce Cost Barriers to Contraception: Issues in Brief.* Alan Guttmacher Institute. www.guttmacher.org/pubs/ib_0799.html.

49. Ibid.

50. Ibid.

## CHAPTER 3: THE GLOBAL AIDS EPIDEMIC: COULD IT HAVE BEEN PREVENTED?

1. Gottlieb, MS, et al. Pneumocystis pneumonia—Los Angeles. *MMWR.* 1981; 30:250–252.

2. Mofenson, LM. Interventions to prevent mother to child HIV transmission: Anti-retroviral prophylaxis trials in resource-rich and resource-limited settings. *UpToDate.* April 26, 2005.

3. Mann, JM. AIDS: Worldwide pandemic. In Gottlieb, MS, et al. (eds.). *Current Topics in AIDS*, Vol. 2. New York: John Wiley and Sons, 1989.

4. McNeil, DG. U.S. urges HIV tests for adults and teenagers. *New York Times.* September 22, 2006. p. A1.

5. Leibowitch, J. *A Strange Virus of Unknown Origin.* New York: Ballantine Books, 1985.

6. Vangroenweghe, D. The earliest cases of human immunodeficiency virus type I group M in Congo-Kinshasa, Rwanda, and Burundi and the origin of acquired immune deficiency syndrome. *Phil Trans Royal Society London.* 2001;356:923–925.

7. Keele, BF, et al. Chimpanzee reservoirs of pandemic and nonpandemic HIV-1. *Science.* 2006;313:523–526.

8. Altman, KL. Chimp virus is linked to HIV. *New York Times.* May 26, 2006.

9. Arno, PS, and Feiden, KL. *Against the Odds: The Story of AIDS Drug Develop-ment, Politics, and Profits.* New York: HarperCollins, 1992.

10. Leibowitch, J. Op cit.

11. Kaiser Family Foundation. *The Global HIV/AIDS Epidemic: A Timeline of Key Milestones.* www.kff.org.

12. Ibid.

13. http://www.gmhc.org/about/timeline.html.

14. Leibowitch, J. Op cit.

15. http://www.ryanwhite.com.

16. Kleinman, S. Transfusion transmitted HIV infection and AIDS. *UpToDate.* August 20, 2004.

17. Epidemiologic notes and reports possible transfusion-associated acquired immune deficiency syndrome, AIDS conference. *MMWR Weekly*. 1982;31:652–654.

18. Simon, M. For Haiti's tourism, the stigma of AIDS is fatal. *New York Times*. November 29, 1983.

19. Jefferson, D. How AIDS changed America. *Newsweek*. May 15, 2006. pp. 36–41.

20. http://www.sfaf.org/aidstimeline/index_all.cfm?type=a.

21. http://www.gmhc.org/about/timeline.html.

22. Cochrane, M. *When AIDS Began: San Francisco and the Making of an Epidemic*. New York: Routledge, 2004.

23. Arno, P, and Keiden, KL. Op cit.

24. Dowdle, WR. The epidemiology of AIDS. *Public Health Reports*. 1983;98:308–312.

25. Conway, G. U.S. capital faces "serious" HIV challenge. *BBC News*. December 1, 2005. www.bbc.co.uk.

26. Leibowitch, J. Op cit.

27. *HIV/AIDS Fact Sheets: The Global Pandemic, the Epidemic in the United States, and Women, Girls, HIV and AIDS*. Elizabeth Glaser Pediatric AIDS Foundation. http://www.pedaids.org.

28. Ibid.

29. Kalb, C, and Murr, A. Battling a black epidemic. *Newsweek*. May 15, 2006. pp. 42–48.

30. The Henry Kaiser Family Foundation. *HIV/AIDS Policy Fact Sheet: The HIV/AIDS Epidemic in the United States*. www.kff.org.

31. Mann, JM. Op cit.

32. Ippolito, G, et al. The changing picture of the HIV/AIDS epidemic. *Annals of New York Academy of Sciences*. 2001;946:1–12.

33. Hooper, C. Critics unimpressed with Reagan's AIDS gambit. United Press International. April 6, 1987.

34. http://www.aidsnews.org.

35. Jefferson, D. Op cit.

36. Beegan, D. Studds says Reagan has shown little concern over AIDS. Associated Press. September 19, 1985.

37. http://www.surgeongeneral.gov/library/history/biokoop.htm.

38. http:www.gmhc.org/abou/timeline.html.

39. Evolution of HIV/AIDS Prevention Programs—United States, 1981–2006. *MMWR*. 2006;55:597–603.

40. http:www.sfaf.org/aidstimeline/index_all.cfm?type+a.

41. Kolata, G. Doctors and patients take AIDS drug trial into their own hands. *New York Times*. March 15, 1988.

42. Boffey, PM. Official blames shortage of staff for delay in testing AIDS drugs. *New York Times*. April 30, 1988.

43. Kolata, G. Patients going underground to buy experimental drugs. *New York Times*. November 4, 1991.

44. Kolata, G. A market for drugs: AIDS patients and their above-ground underground. *New York Times*. July 10, 1988.

45. Approval of AZT. *Public Health Service*. March 20, 1987. www.fda.gov/bbs/topics/NEWS/NEW00217.html.

46. Rimmerman, CA. *ACT UP*. 1998. http://www.thebody.com.

47. ADAP Fact Sheet. http://www.bah.hrsa.gov/programs/factsheet/adap.

48. NASTAD. *The ADAP Watch*. June 15, 2006. www.nastad.org.

49. Walensky, RP, et al. The survival benefits of AIDS treatment in the United States. *J Infectious Dis*. 2006;194:11–19.

50. Pomerantz, RJ, and Horn, DL. Twenty years of therapy for HIV-1 infection. *Nature Med*. 2003;9:867–873.

51. Schwartlander, B, et al. The 10-year struggle to provide antiretroviral treatment to people with HIV in the developing world. *Lancet*. 2006;368:541–546.

52. Kellerman, S, et al. Changes in HIV and AIDS in the United States: Entering the third decade. *Current HIV/AIDS Reports*. 2004;1:153–158.

53. Kalichman, SX (ed.). *Positive Prevention: Reducing HIV Transmission among People Living with HIV/AIDS*. New York: Kluwer Academic/Plenum Publishers, 2005.

54. Kim, JY, and Farmer, P. AIDS in 2006—moving toward one world, one hope? *New Engl J Med*. 2006;355:645–647.

55. Cowley, G. The life of a virus hunter. *Newsweek*. May 15, 2006. pp. 63–65.

56. www.gmhc.org/timeline.

57. McNeil, DG. Op cit.

58. Buve, A, et al. The spread and effect of HIV-1 infection in Sub-Saharan Africa. *Lancet*. 2002;359:2011–2017.

59. UNAIDS. *Basic Facts About the AIDS Epidemic and Its Impact*. November 2004. http://www.unaids.org.

60. The Henry J. Kaiser Family Foundation. *HIV/AIDS Policy Fact Sheet: HIV/AIDS Epidemic in Sub-Saharan Africa*. October 2005. www.kff.org.

61. UNAIDS. *2006 Report on the Global AIDS Epidemic*. 2006. www.unaids.org.

62. *HIV/AIDS in South Africa*. www.southafricainfo.org.

63. Pape, J, and Johnson, WD. AIDS in Haiti: 1982–1992. *Clin Infect Dis*. 1993;17:S341–S345.

64. Ghys, PD, et al. Growing in silence: Selected regions and countries with expanding HIV/AIDS epidemics. *AIDS*. 2003;17:S45–S50.

65. UNAIDS and WHO. *AIDS Epidemic Update: Special Report on HIV Prevention*. December 2005. http://www.unaids.org.

66. Pais, P. HIV and India: Looking into the abyss. *Tropical Med and Internatl Health*. 1996;1:295–304.

67. Cohen, J. HIV/AIDS in China. Poised for a takeoff? *Science*. 2004;304(5676):1430–1432.

68. He, N, and Detels, R. The HIV epidemic in China: History, response, and challenge. *Cell Research*. 2005;15:825–832.

69. Phoolcharoen, W. HIV/AIDS prevention in Thailand: Success and challenges. *Science*. 1998;280(5371):1873–1874.

70. Quinn, TC. The global human immunodeficiency virus pandemic. *UpToDate*. September 17, 2004.

71. UNAIDS. *2004 Report on the Global AIDS Epidemic: Executive Summary*. June 2004. http://www.unaids.org.

72. UNAIDS. *International Programmes, Initiatives, and Funding Issues*. June 2005. http://www.unaids.org.

73. D'Adesky, AC. *Moving Mountains: The Race to Treat Global AIDS*. New York: Verso, 2004.

74. Kazmin, A. Thai victory on AIDS drug patent paves the way for others. *Financial Times*. February 20, 2004.

75. Teixeira, PR, et al. Antiretroviral treatment in resource-poor settings: The Brazilian experience. *AIDS*. 2004;18:S5–S7.

76. Berkman, A, et al. A critical analysis of the Brazilian response to HIV/AIDS: Lessons learned for controlling and mitigating the epidemic in developing countries. *Am J Public Health*. 2005;95:1162–1172.

77. Feachem, RGA, and Sabot, OJ. An examination of the global fund at 5 years. *Lancet*. 2006;368:537–540.

78. The Henry J. Kaiser Family Foundation. *HIV/AIDS Policy Fact Sheet: HIV/AIDS in India*. September 2005. www.kff.org.

79. Dugger, CW. Clinton makes up for lost time in battling AIDS. *New York Times*. August 29, 2006.

80. Clinton cuts a deal for kids with AIDS. Associated Press. November 30, 2006.

81. Basu, P. South Africa to distribute AIDS drug. *Nat Med*. 2003;9:1098.

82. *The '3 by 5' Initiative*. www.who.int.

83. *The State of Global Research*. http://www.iavi.org.

84. Solomon, J. Sides differ over failure to develop AIDS vaccine. *Hartford Courant*. December 26, 2005. p. A7.

85. http://www.hivvaccineenterprise.org/plan/1.html.

86. Burkhalter, H. The politics of AIDS: Engaging conservative activities. *Foreign Affairs*. 2004. www.foreignaffairs.org.

87. Kaiser Family Foundation. *Survey of Americans on HIV/AIDS*. www.kff.org.

## CHAPTER 4: THE STEM CELL CONTROVERSY: NAVIGATING A SEA OF ETHICS, POLITICS, AND SCIENCE

1. Usdin, S. Ethical issues associated with pluripotent stem cells. In Chiu, A, and Rao, MS (eds.). *Human Embryonic Stem Cells*. Totowa, NJ: Humana Press, 2003. pp. 3–26.

2. Fischbach, GD, and Fischbach, RL. Stem cells: Science, policy, and ethics. *J Clin Invest*. 2004;114:1364–1370.

3. Bongso, A, and Lee, EH. Stem cells: Their definition, classification, and sources. In Bongso, A, and Lee, EH (eds.). *Stem Cells: From Bench to Bedside*. Hackensack, NJ: World Scientific, 2005. pp. 1–13.

4. Prosper, F, and Verfaillie, CM. Human pluripotent stem cells from bone marrow. In Chiu, A, and Rao, MS (eds.). *Human Embryonic Stem Cells*. Totowa, NJ: Humana Press, 2003. pp. 89–112.

5. Kiessling, AA, and Anderson, SC. *Human Embryonic Stem Cell: An Introduction to the Science and Therapeutic Potential*. Boston: Jones and Bartlett, 2003.

6. Parson, A. *Proteus Effect: Stem Cells and Their Promise in Medicine*. Washington, DC: Joseph Henry Press, 2004.

7. Van Bekkum, DW. Bone marrow transplantation. *Transplant Proc*. 1977;9:147–154.

8. Usdin, S. Op cit.

9. Thompson, JA, et al. Embryonic stem cell lines derived from human blastocysts. *Science*. 1998;282:1145–1147. Shamblott, MJ, et al. Derivation of pluripotent stem cells from cultured human primordial germ cells. *Proc Natl Acad Sci USA*. 1998;95:13726–13731.

10. Vogel, G. Breakthrough of the year: Capturing the promise of youth. *Science*. 1999;286(5448):2238–2239.

11. Wilmut, I, and Paterson, LA. Stem cells and cloning. In Sell, S (ed.). *Stem Cells Handbook*. Totowa, NJ: Humana Press, 2004.

12. Horb, ME, et al. Experimental conversion of liver to pancreas. *Current Biology*. 2003;13:105–115.

13. Bongso, A, and Lee, EH. Op cit.

14. Parson, A. Op cit.

15. Hwang, SW, et al. Patient-specific embryonic stem cells derived from human SCNT blastocysts. *Science*. 2005;308(5729):1777–1183.

16. Cyranoski, D. South Korean scandal rocks stem cell community. *Natl Med*. 2006;12:4.

17. O'Brien, TA, et al. No longer a biological waste product: Umbilical cord blood. *Med J Aust*. 2006;184:407–410.

18. Young, MJ. Stem cells in the mammalian eye: A tool for retinal repair. *APMIS*. 2005;113:845–857.

19. McDonald, JW, et al. Transplanted embryonic stem cells survive, differentiate and promote recovery in injured rat spinal cord. *Natl Med*. 1999;5:1410–1412.

20. Wichterle, H, et al. Directed differentiation of embryonic stem cells into motor neurons. *Cell*. 2002;110:385–397.

21. *CDC Statistics*. June 20, 2006. www.cdc.gov/nchs/fastats/lcod.htm.

22. Kehat, I, et al. Electromechanical integration of cardiomyocytes derived from human embryonic stem cells. *Natl Biotechnol*. 2004;22:1282–1289.

23. Fraidenreich, D, et al. Rescue of cardiac defects in ID knockout embryos by injection of embryonic stem cells. *Science*. 2004;306(5694):247–252.

24. Fraidenreich, D, and Benezra, R. Embryonic stem cells prevent developmental cardiac defects in mice. *Nature Clin Practice Cardiovasc Med*. 2006;3:S14–S17.

25. Schmidt, D, et al. Living patches engineered from human umbilical cord derived fibroblasts and endothelial progenitor cells. *Eur J Cardiothorac Surg*. 2005;27:795–800.

26. Walter, BL, and Vitek, JL. Surgical treatment for Parkinson's disease. *Lancet Neurol*. 2004;3:719–728.

27. Takagi, Y, et al. Dopaminergic neurons generated from monkey embryonic stem cells function in a Parkinson primate model. *J Clin Invest*. 2005;115:102–109.

28. Boyle, JP, et al. Projection of diabetes burden through 2050. *Diabetes Care*. 2001;24:1936–1940.

29. www.wisctechnology.com/article.php?id-2340.

30. Green, RM. *The Human Embryo Research Debates: Bioethics in the Vortex of Controversy*. New York: Oxford University Press, 2001.

31. Chung, Y, et al. Embryonic and extraembryonic stem cell lines derived from single mouse blastomeres. *Nature*. 2006;439:216–219.

32. Meissner, A, and Jaenisch, R. Generation of nuclear transfer-derived pluripotent ES cells from cloned cdx2-deficient blastocysts. *Nature*. 2006; 439:212–215.

33. Studies may calm stem cell qualms. Associated Press. October 16, 2005.

34. Wade, N. Stem cells with ethics. *New York Times*. October 16, 2005.

35. Bush's stem cell policy received with mixed emotions. www.lifesite.net.

36. Perkins, T. Embryonic stem cell studies raise questions, not cures. *Washington Update*. October 16, 2005.

37. Ritter, M. Studies show new ways to get stem cells. Associated Press. October 16, 2005.

38. Stem cell without embryo loss. *New York Times.* August 26, 2006. p. A35.

39. Cook, G. Stem cell method preserves embryo; Mass. lab hopes to end standoff. *Boston Globe.* August 24, 2006. p. A1.

40. Sutherland, W. *Embryonic Stem Cell Research: Overcoming the Ethical Barriers.* Ezine@rticles. www.ezinearticles.com.

41. Bonnicksen, AL. *Crafting a Cloning Policy: From Dolly to Stem Cells.* Washington, DC: Georgetown University Press, 2002. pp. 77–79.

42. Fischbach, GD, and Fischbach, RL. Op cit.

43. *The Need for Guidelines to Govern Research Using Pluripotent Stem Cells.* www.nih.gov/news/stemcell/index.htm.

44. Wertz, DC. Embryo and stem cell research in the United States: History and politics. *Gene Therapy.* 2002;9:674–678.

45. Casell, JH. Lengthening the stem: Allowing federally funded researchers to derive human pluripotent stem cells from embryos. *Univ Mich J Law Reform.* 2001;34:547–572.

46. *White Paper: Alternative Sources of Pluripotent Stem Cells.* Washington, DC: President's Council on Bioethics, 2005.

47. NIH Budget Office. April 16, 2006.

48. Stevens, D. Embryonic stem cell research: Will President Bush's limitation on federal funding put the United States at a disadvantage? A comparison between U.S. and international law. *Houston J Internatl Law.* 2003;25:623–653.

49. Panetta, J, et al. California Stem Cell Research and Cures Act: What to expect from stem cell research. *J Biolaw Bus.* 2005;8:3–12.

50. http://www.state.nj.us/scitech/stem_intro.html.

51. Most Americans support aggressive stem cell research, says a new nationwide poll. http://forthemedia.uthouston.edu/newsrreleases/nr2004/zogby.html.

52. Rudoren, J. Stem cell work gets states' aid after Bush veto. *New York Times.* July 25, 2006. p. A1.

53. Kurtzman, L. Schwarzenegger funds stem cell research. Associated Press. July 21, 2006.

## CHAPTER 5: MARIJUANA AS MEDICINE: SCIENCE VERSUS POLITICS

1. *UK Cannabis Campaigners' Guide.* http://www.ccguide.org.uk.

2. http://wikipedia.org/wiki/hemp.

3. Institute of Medicine. *Marijuana and Medicine: Assessing the Science Base.* Washington, DC: National Academy of Sciences, 1999.

4. Mechoulam, R (ed.). *Marijuana: Chemistry, Pharmacology, Metabolism, and Clinical Effects.* New York: Academic Press, 1973.

5. Adams, IB, and Marion, BR. Cannabis: Pharmacology and toxicology in animals and humans. *Addiction.* 1996;91:1585–1614.

6. Herkenham, M, et al. Cannabinoid receptor localization in the brain. *Proc Natl Acad Sci USA.* 1990;87:1932–1936.

7. Institute of Medicine. Op cit.

8. *History of Marijuana as Medicine: 2037 B.C. to Present.* www.medical marijuanaprocon.org.

9. http://www.wikipedia.org/wiki/medical_marijuana.

10. Herer, J. *The Emperor Wears No Clothes.* www.jackherer.com.

11. Ibid.

12. Ibid.

13. *UK Cannabis Campaigners' Guide.* Op cit.

14. The British Advisory Committee on Drug Dependence Cannabis. *Wooten Report.* 1968.

15. *Cannabis Use in the U.S.: Implications for Policy.* Newark, DE: University of Delaware. Center for Drug and Alcohol Studies; June 12, 1995.

16. *Cannabis Use in the U.S.: Implications for Policy.* University of Delaware. Op cit.

17. *UK Cannabis Campaigners' Guide.* Op cit.

18. www.medicalmarijuanaprocon.org.

19. *Provision of Marijuana and Other Compounds for Scientific Research.* Washington, DC: NIDA, 1998.

20. U.S. Dept of Justice, Drug Enforcement Agency. *In the Matter of Marijuana Rescheduling Petition.* Docket #86-22. September 6, 1988. p. 57.

21. W. Armentano, P. The fight for medical marijuana. *Liberty.* January 1998; XI,3:31–32.

22. Institute of Medicine. Op cit.

23. Kassirer, JP. Federal foolishness and marijuana. *New Engl J Med.* 1997;336:366–367.

24. Supreme Court rules against medical marijuana. *WebMD Medical News.* June 6, 2005.

25. Carter, GT, et al. Medicinal cannabis: Rational guidelines for dosing. *Drugs.* 2004;7:464–470.

26. Institute of Medicine. Op cit.

27. Herming, RI, Hooker, WD, Jones, RT. Tetrahydrocannabinol content and differences in marijuana smoking behavior. *Psychopharmacology.* 1986;90:160–162.

28. Tashkin, DP. Pulmonary complications of smoked substance abuse. *West J Med.* 1990;152:525–530.

29. Zhang, ZF, Morgenstern, H, Spitz, MR, et al. Marijuana use and increased risk of squamous cell carcinoma of the head and neck. *Cancer Epidemiology, Biomarkers, and Prev.* 1999;6:1071–1078.

30. Tashkin, DP. Op cit.

31. Sridhar, KS, et al. Possible role of marijuana smoking as a carcinogen in the development of lung cancer at a young age. *J Psychoactive Drugs.* 1994;26:285–288.

32. Mittleman, MA, et al. Triggering myocardial infarction by marijuana. *Circulation.* 2001;103:2805–2809.

33. Brook, JS, et al. The effect of early marijuana use on later anxiety and depressive symptoms. *NYS Psychologist.* January 2001. pp. 35–39.

34. Green, BE, and Itter, C. Marijuana use and depression. *J Health Soc Behavior.* 2000;41:40–49.

35. Brook, JS, Cohen, P, and Brook, DW. Longitudinal study of co-occurring psychiatric disorders and substance use. *J Acad Child and Adoles Psychol.* 1998;37:322–330.

36. Pope, HG, and Yrgolun-Todd, D. The residual cognitive effects of heavy marijuana use in college students. *JAMA.* 1996;272:521–527.

37. Kouri, EM, Pope, HG, and Lukas, SE. Changes in aggressive behavior during withdrawal from long-term marijuana use. *Psychopharmacology.* 1999;143:395–404.

38. Campbell, FA, et al. Are cannabinoids an effective and safe treatment option in the management of pain? A qualitative systematic review. *BMJ*. 2001;323:13–16.

39. Ware, MA, et al. Cannabis use among patients with HIV/AIDS: patterns and prevalence of use. *J Cannabis Therapy*. 2003;3:3–15.

40. Sallan, SE, Zinberg, NE, ad Frei, E. Antiemetic effect of delta-9-tetrahydrocanna-binol in patients receiving cancer chemotherapy. *New Engl J Med*. 1975;293:795–797.

41. Marijuana eases HIV-related nerve pain. *Reuters Health*. February 12, 2004.

42. Svendson, KB, Jensen, TS, and Bach, FW. Does the cannabinoid dronabinol reduce central pain in multiple sclerosis? Randomized double blind placebo controlled crossover trial. *BMJ*. 2004;329:257–258.

43. Hepler, RS, and Frank, IR. Marihuana smoking and intraocular pressure (Letter). *JAMA*. 1971;217:1392.

44. Green, K. Marijuana smoking vs. cannabinoids for glaucoma therapy. *Arch Ophthalmol*. 1998;116:1433–1437.

45. National Eye Institute. *The Use of Marijuana for Glaucoma: Statement of the National Eye Institute of the National Institutes of Health*. February 18, 1997.

46. Pryce, G, et al. Cannabinoids inhibit neurodegeneration in models of multiple sclerosis. *Brain*. 2003;136:2191–2202.

47. Wade, DT, et al. A preliminary controlled study to determine whether whole-plant canabis extracts can improve intractable neurogenic symptoms. *Clin Rehabil*. 2003;17:21–29.

48. Goodin, D. Marijuana and multiple sclerosis. *Lancet Neurol*. 2004;3:79–80.

49. Corey, S. Recent developments in the therapeutic potential of cannabinoids. *PR Health Sci J*. 2005;24:19–26.

50. Killestein, J, Uitdehaag, BMJ, and Polman, CH. Cannabinoids in multiple sclerosis: Do they have a therapeutic role? *Drugs*. 2004;64:1–11.

51. Zajicek, J, et al. Cannabinoids for treatment of spasticity and other symptoms related to multiple sclerosis (CAMS Study): Multicentre randomized placebo-controlled trial. *Lancet*. 2003;362:1517–1526.

52. Woolridge, E, et al. Cannabis use in HIV for pain and other medical symptoms. *J Pain and Symptom Mgmt*. 2005;29:358–367.

53. Plasse, TF, et al. Recent clinical experience with dronabinol. *Pharmacol Biochem Behav*. 1991;40:695–700.

54. Abrams, D, et al. Short term effects of cannabinoids in patients with HIV-1 infection. *Ann Internal Med*. 2003;139:258–266.

55. CNN/Time Poll. Nov 4, 2002.

56. Wolfe, E. 75 percent in AARP poll back medical marijuana use. Associated Press. December 19, 2004.

57. Doblin, R, and Kleiman, MAR. Marijuana as anti-emetic medicine: A survey of oncologists' experiences and attitudes. *J Clin Oncol*. 1991;9:1275–1280.

## CHAPTER 6: THE QUINTESSENTIAL CATCH-22: THE U.S. APPROACH TO NEEDLE EXCHANGE IN HIV AIDS PREVENTION

1. Centers for Disease Control and Prevention. Update: Syringe exchange programs, United States, 2002. *MMWR*. 2005;54:673–676.

2. Paone, D, et al. Syringe exchange in the United States, 1996: A national profile. *Am J Public Health*. 1999;89:43–46.

3. Human Rights Watch. *Injecting Reason, Human Rights, and HIV Prevention for Injection Drug Users, California: A Case Study.* September 2003; Vol 15, No 2 (G).

4. American Rhetoric. Ronald Reagan: First Inaugural Address. Retrieved on August 20, 2005 from http://www.americanrhetoric.com/speeches/rreagandfirstinaugural. html.

5. *Confronting AIDS: Directions for Public Health, Health Care, and Research.* Washington, DC: National Academy of Sciences, 1987.

6. Scheer, R. We are not lepers: AIDS stigma hampering a solution. *Los Angeles Times.* November 28, 1986.

7. *AIDS Knowledge and Attitudes for May and June 1988: Provisional Data from the National Health Interview Survey.* Hyattsville, MD: U.S. Department of Health and Human Services, National Center for Health Statistics, 1988.

8. *AIDS Surveillance Trends.* www.cdc.gov/hiv/graphics/trends/html.

9. Fernando, D. *AIDS and Intravenous Drug Use: The Influence of Morality, Politics, Social Science, and Race in the Making of a Tragedy.* Westport, CT: Praeger, 1993.

10. Centers for Disease Control and Prevention. *HIV/AIDS Surveillance Report.* http://www.cdc.gov/hiv/stats/hasrlink.HTM.

11. Centers for Disease Control and Prevention. HIV diagnoses among injection drug users in states with HIV surveillance: 25 states, 1994–2000. *MMWR.* 2003;52:634–636.

12. Lane, S, Stryker, J, and Smith, M. *Needle Exchange: A Brief History.* 1993. http://www.aegis.com/law/journals/1993/HKFNE009.html.

13. Van Ameijden, E. The harm reduction approach and risk factors for human immunodeficiency virus (HIV) seroconversion in injection drug users. *Amer J Epi.* 1992;136:236–242.

14. Normand, J, et al. Panel on Needle Exchange and Bleach Distribution Programs. *Preventing HIV Transmission: The Role of Sterile Needles and Bleach.* Washington, DC: National Academies Press, 1995.

15. Bennett, W. Should drugs be legalized? In Schaler, J (ed.). *Drugs: Should We Legalize, Decriminalize, or Deregulate?* Amherst, NY: Prometheus Books, 1997. pp. 63–67.

16. U.S. Department of Health and Human Services, Office of Applied Studies. Heroin Abuse in the United States. http://www.oas.samhsa.gov/NHSDA/Treatan/ treana12.htm#E10E35.

17. National Commission on AIDS. *The Twin Epidemics of Substance Use and HIV.* Washington, DC: Commission on AIDS, 1991.

18. *Needle Exchange Programs: Research Suggests Promise as an AIDS Prevention Strategy.* Washington, DC: General Accounting Office, 1993.

19. Lovett, D. A metabolic basis for drug dependence. *Canadian Psychiatric Association Journal.* 1974;19:487–494.

20. Schilit, R, and Gomberg, E. *Drugs and Behavior: A Sourcebook for the Helping Professions.* London: Sage, 1991.

21. Wikler, A. Conditioning factors in opiate addiction and relapse. In Wilner, D, and Kassebaum, G (eds.). *Narcotics.* New York: McGraw-Hill, 1965.

22. Needle exchange programs: Are they effective? *Office of National Drug Control Policy Bulletin.* 1992;7:1–7.

23. Wren, C. White House drug and AIDS advisers differ on needle exchange. *New York Times.* March 23, 1998. p. A10.

24. Hart, GJ, et al. Evaluation of needle exchange in central London: Behaviour change and anti-HIV status over one year. *AIDS*. 1989;3:261–265.

25. Van den Hoek, J, Van Haastrecht, H, and Coutinho, R. Risk reduction among intravenous drug users in Amsterdam under the influence of AIDS. *Am J Public Health*. 1989;79:1355–1357.

26. Vlahov, D, et al. Reductions in high-risk drug use behaviors among participants in the Baltimore needle exchange program. *Journal of Acquired Immunodeficiency Syndromes*. 1997;16:400–406.

27. Bluthenthal, R, et al. The effect of syringe exchange use on high-risk injection drug users: A cohort study. *AIDS*. 2000;14:605–611.

28. Des Jarlais, D, et al. Maintaining low HIV seroprevalence in populations of injecting drug users. *JAMA*. 1995;274:1226–1231.

29. Hagan, H, et al. Reduced risk of hepatitis B and hepatitis C among injection drug users in the Tacoma syringe exchange program. *Am J Public Health*. 1995;85:1531–1537.

30. Brooner, R, et al. Drug abuse treatment success among needle exchange participants. *Public Health Reports*. 1995;113:129–139.

31. Allen, D, Onorato, I, and Green, T. HIV Infection in intravenous drug users entering drug treatment, United States, 1988–1989. *Am J Public Health*. 1992;82:541–546.

32. Gibson, D, Flynn, N, and Perales, D. Effectiveness of syringe exchange programs in reducing HIV risk behavior and HIV seroconversion among injecting drug users. *AIDS*. 2001;15:1329–1341.

33. Commonwealth Department of Health and Aging. *Return on Investment in Needle and Syringe Programmes in Australia*. 2002.http://www.health.gov.au/internet/wcms/Publishing.nsf/Content/health-pubhlth-publicat-document-roireport-cnt.html.

34. Neergaard, L. Advisers on AIDS urge U.S. spending on needles. Associated Press. March 17, 1998.

35. AIDS Action. *Needle Exchange Facts*. 2001. www.aidsaction.org/legislation/pdf/Policy_Facts-Needle_Exchange2.pdf.

36. Law, Policy, and Public Health at Temple University's Beasley School of Law. *Nonprescription Access*. http://www.temple.edu/lawschool/aidspolicy/50statesataglance.htm.

37. Jarlais, D, et al. 2000 *National Syringe Exchange Survey*. http://www.opiate addictionrx.info/survey2000.

38. Prince, B. *Law Enforcement and Risky Injection Behavior: Preliminary Ethnographic Findings and Fieldnotes*. www.hrw.org/reports/2003.

39. Sternberg, S. Clinton "wrong" on needle swaps. *USA Today*. July 11, 2002.

## CHAPTER 7: BLEAK HOUSE AND BEYOND: HOW TUBERCULOSIS CONTROL GOT SIDE-TRACKED

1. Coker, R. Lessons from New York's tuberculosis epidemic. *BMJ*. 1998;317:616.

2. Ruggiero, D. A glimpse at the colorful history of TB: Its toll and its effect on the U.S. and the world. *TB Notes Newsletter*. No. 1. Atlanta: Centers for Disease Control and Prevention, Division of Tuberculosis Elimination, 2000.

3. World Health Organization. *WHO Global Tuberculosis Control: Surveillance, Planning, Financing*. Geneva: WHO, 2005. Report WHO/HTM/TB 2005.

4. Markel, H. TB: The epidemic to truly worry about. *The Globalist.* March 25, 2004.

5. *Tuberculosis: A Global Emergency.* Princeton Project 55, Inc. Tuberculosis Initiative. April 1999.

6. *WHO Research for Action: Understanding and Controlling Tuberculosis in India.* Geneva: WHO, 2000.

7. Raviglione, MC, and Nunn, P. Epidemiology of tuberculosis. In Zumla, A, et al. (eds.). *AIDS and Respiratory Medicine.* London: Chapman and Hill, 1997. pp. 117–141.

8. Fairchild, AL, and Oppenheimer, GM. Public health nihilism vs. pragmatism: History, politics, and the control of tuberculosis. *Am J Public Health.* 1998;88:1105–1111.

9. Waksman, SA, Geiger, WB, and Reynolds, DM. Strain specificity and production of antibiotic substances. *Proc Natl Acad Sci USA.* 1946;32:112–120.

10. *A Strategic Plan for the Elimination of Tuberculosis in the United States.* Atlanta: Centers for Disease Control and Prevention, 1989.

11. *Reported Tuberculosis in the United States, 2001.* www.cdcnpin.org.

12. Advisory Council for the Elimination of Tuberculosis. CDC tuberculosis elimination revisited: Obstacles, opportunities, and a renewed commitment. *MMWR.* 1999; 48(No. RR-9):1–13.

13. National action plan to combat multidrug-resistant tuberculosis. Atlanta: Centers for Disease Control and Prevention. *MMWR.* June 19, 1992. www.cdc.gov/mmwr/preview/mmwrhtml.

14. Institute of Medicine. *Ending Neglect: The Elimination of Tuberculosis in the U.S.* Washington, DC: National Academy Press, 2000.

15. *Reported Tuberculosis in the United States, 2001.* www.cdcnpin.org.

16. McKenna, MT, et al. The fall after the rise: Tuberculosis in the United States, 1991 through 1994. *Am J Public Health.* 1998;88:1059–1063.

17. Sotir, MJ, et al. Tuberculosis in the inner city: Impact of a continuing epidemic in the 1990s. *Clin Infect Dis.* 1999;29:1138–1144.

18. World Health Organization. *2001: Global Tuberculosis Control.* Geneva: WHO, 2001. Report WHO/CDS/TB 2001.

19. *Stop TB Partnership: Report on the Meeting of the Second Ad Hoc Committee on the TB Epidemic.* Geneva: WHO, 2004. WHO/HTM/STB/2004.

20. Gates triples TB eradication funds. *The Independent.* June 15, 2006.

21. Frieden, TR, et al. Tuberculosis. *Lancet.* 2003;362:887–899.

22. Blumberg, HM. Treatment of latent tuberculosis infection. Back to the beginning. *Clin Infect Dis.* 2004;39:1772–1775.

23. Borgdorff, MW, et al. Interventions to reduce tuberculosis mortality and transmission in low and middle income countries. *Bull World Health Organ.* 2002;80:217–227.

24. Blumberg, HM, et al. Update on the treatment of tuberculosis and latent tuberculosis infection. *JAMA.* 2005;293:2776–2784.

25. Dye, C, et al. Evolution of tuberculosis control and prospects for reducing tuberculosis incidence, prevalence, and deaths globally. *JAMA.* 2005;293:2767–2775.

26. World Health Organization. *Global TB Control Report.* 2003.

27. American Thoracic Society, CDC and Infectious Disease Society of America. Treatment of tuberculosis. *MMWR.* 2003;52(No. RR-11):1–74.

28. CDC's Response to Ending Neglect. www.cdc.gov/nchstp/tb/pubs/IOM/iomresponse/execsummary.htm.

29. *Virtually Untreatable TB Finding*. www.news.bbc.co.uk.

## CHAPTER 8: SCIENCE, POLITICS, AND THE REGULATION OF DIETARY SUPPLEMENTS

1. Eastman, P. Strike three for dietary supplements? *AARP Bulletin*. December 13, 2006.

2. Dietary Supplement Health and Education Act of 1994. Pub Law No 103-417, 108 Stat 4325 (October 25, 1994).

3. Bent, S, and Ko, R. Commonly used herbal medicines in the United States: A review. *Am J Medicine*. 2004;116:478–485.

4. Eisenberg, DM, et al. Unconventional medicine in the United States. *New Engl J Med*. 1993;328:246–252.

5. Eisenberg, DM, et al. Trends in alternative medicine use in the United States, 1990–1997: Results of a follow up national survey. *JAMA*. 1998;280:1569–1575.

6. Stein, R. Alternative remedies gaining popularity. *Washington Post*. September 5, 2004. p. A1.

7. Kelly, JP, et al. Recent trends in use of herbal and other natural products. *Arch Intern Med*. 2005;165:281–286.

8. *Dietary Supplements: A Framework for Evaluating Safety*. Washington, DC: Institute of Medicine, 2004.

9. Blendon, RJ, et al. Americans' views on the use and regulation of dietary supplements. *Arch Intern Med*. 2001;161:805–810.

10. Kaufman, DW, et al. Recent patterns of medication use in the ambulatory adult population of the United States: The Slone survey. *JAMA*. 2002;287:337–344.

11. Palmer, ME, and Howland, MA. Herbals and dietary supplements. In Ford, M, et al. (eds.). *Clinical Toxicology*. Philadelphia: Saunders, 2001. pp. 316–331.

12. DeSmet, RAGM. Health risks of herbal remedies: An update. *Clin Pharmacol and Therapeutics*. 2004;76:1–17.

13. Samenuk, D, et al. Adverse cardiovascular events temporally associated with ma huang, an herbal source of ephedrine. *Mayo Clinic Proc*. 2002;77:12–16.

14. Stampfer, MJ, et al. Vitamin E consumption and the risk of coronary heart disease in women. *New Engl J Med*. 1993;328:1444–1449.

15. Rimm, EB. Vitamin E consumption and the risk of coronary health disease in men. *New Engl J Med*. 1993;328:1450–1456.

16. Rimm, EB, and Stampfer, MJ. Antioxidants for vascular disease. *Med Clin North America*. 2000;84:239–249.

17. Lee, IM, et al. Vitamin E in the primary prevention of cardiovascular disease and cancer. The Women's Health Study: A randomized controlled trial. *JAMA*. 2005; 294:56–65.

18. Pham, DQ. Vitamin E supplementation in cardiovascular disease and cancer prevention: Part 1. *Annals of Pharmacotherapy*. 2005;39:1870–1878.

19. Petersen, RC, et al. Vitamin E and donepezil for the treatment of mild cognitive impairment. *New Engl J Med*. 2005;352:2379–2388.

20. Zhang, S, et al. Dietary carotenoids and vitamins A, C, and E and risk of breast cancer. *J Natl Cancer Inst*. 1999;91:547–556.

21. Jacobs, EJ, et al. Vitamin C and vitamin E supplement use and colorectal cancer mortality in a large American Cancer Society cohort. *Cancer Epidemiol Biomarkers Prev*. 2001;10:17–23.

22. Alpha-Tocopherol, Beta Carotene Cancer Prevention (ATBC) Trial. www.cancer.gov/newscenter/pressreleases/ATBCfollowup.

23. The effect of vitamin E and beta carotene on the incidence of lung cancer and other cancers in male smokers: The alpha-tocopherol, beta carotene cancer prevention study group. *New Engl J Med*. 1994;330:1029–1035.

24. Omenn, GS, et al. Effects of a combination of beta carotene and vitamin A on lung cancer and cardiovascular disease. *New Engl J Med*. 1996;334:1150–1155.

25. Blot, WJ, et al. Nutrition intervention trials in Linxian China: Supplementation with specific vitamin/mineral combinations, cancer incidence, and disease-specific mortality in the general population. *J Natl Cancer Inst*. 1993;85:1483–1492.

26. Lee, IM, et al. Beta-carotene supplementation and incidence of cancer and cardiovascular disease: The Women's Health Study. *J Natl Cancer Inst*. 1999;91:2102–2106.

27. Cook, NR, et al. Effects of beta carotene supplementation on cancer incidence by baseline characteristics in the Physicians' Health Study (United States). *Cancer Causes Control*. 2000;11:617–626.

28. Zhang, S, et al. Op cit.

29. Bazzano, LA, et al. Effect of folic acid supplementation on risk of cardiovascular diseases. A meta-analysis of randomized controlled trials. *JAMA*. 2006;296:2720–2726.

30. Homocysteine lowering with folic acid and B vitamins in vascular disease. The Heart Outcomes Prevention Evaluation (HOPE) 2 Investigators. *New Engl J Med*. 2006;354:1567–1577.

31. McAlindon, TE, et al. Glucosamine and chondroitin for treatment of osteoarthritis: A systematic quality assessment and meta-analysis. *JAMA*. 2000;283:1469–1475.

32. Barrett, BP, et al. Treatment of the common cold with unrefined echinacea. A randomized, double-blind, placebo-controlled trial. *Ann Intern Med*. 2002;137:939–946.

33. Grimm, W, and Muller, H. A randomized clinical trial on the effect of fluid extract of Echinacea purpurea on the incidence and severity of colds and respiratory infections. *Ann J Med*. 1999;106:138–143.

34. Taylor, JA, et al. Efficacy and safety of Echinacea in treating upper respiratory tract infections in children. *JAMA*. 2006;290:2824–2830.

35. Williams, JW, et al. A systematic review of newer pharmacotherapies for depression in adults: Evidence report summary. *Ann Intern Med*. 2000;132:743–756.

36. Gaster, B, and Holroyd, J. St. John's wort for depression: A systematic review. *Arch Intern Med*. 2000;160:152–160.

37. Linde, K, and Mulrow, CD. St. John's wort for depression. *Cochrane Review*. Oxford: Cochrane Library. Issue 3, 2002.

38. Phillipp, M, Kohnen, R, and Hiller, KO. Hypericum extract versus imipramine or placebo in patients with moderate depression: Randomised multicentre study of treatment for eight weeks. *BMJ*. 1999;319:1534–1538.

39. Shelton, RC, et al. Effectiveness of St. John's wort in major depression. A randomized control trial. *JAMA*. 2001;285:1978–1986.

40. Effect of Hypericum perforatu (St. John's wort) in major depressive disorders: A randomized clinical trial. Hypericum Depression Trial Study Group. *JAMA*. 2002;287:1807–1814.

41. Nair, KS, et al. DHEA in elderly women and DHEA or testosterone in elderly men. *New Engl J Med.* 2006;355:1647–1659.

42. Muller, M, et al. Effects of dehydroepiandrosterone and atamestane supplementation on frailty in elderly men. *Med J Clin Endocrinol Metab.* (in press).

43. Stevinson, C, Pittler, MH, and Ernest, E. Garlic for treating hypercholesterolemia. A meta-analysis of randomized clinical trials. *Ann Intern Med.* 2000;133:420–429.

44. Ernest, E, and Pittler, MH. Ginkgo biloba extract for dementia: A systematic review of double-blind, placebo-controlled trials. *Clin Drug Invest.* 1999;17:301–308.

45. Wilt, TJ, et al. Saw palmetto extracts for treatment of benign prostatic hyperplasia: A systematic review. *JAMA.* 1998;280:1604–1609.

46. *Dietary Supplements: Background Information.* Office of Dietary Supplements. National Institutes of Health. www.ods.od.nih.gov/factsheets/dietarysupplements.asp.

47. Ibid.

48. Morris, CA, and Avorn, J. Internet marketing of herbal products. *JAMA.* 2003; 290,11:1505–1509.

49. Ibid.

50. Fox, S, and Rainie, L. *Vital Decisions: How Internet Users Decide What Information to Trust When They or Their Loved Ones Are Sick.* Washington, DC: Pew Internet and American Life Project, 2002.

51. *Adverse Event Reporting for Dietary Supplements: An Inadequate Safety Valve.* Washington, DC: Office of the Inspector General, 2001. OE1-01-00180.

52. DeSmet, RAGM. Op cit.

53. Kressmann, S, Muller, WE, and Blume, HH. Pharmaceutical quality of different ginkgo biloba brands. *J Pharm Pharmacol.* 2002;54:661–669.

54. Bent, S, and Ko, R. Op cit.

55. Ross, EA, et al. Lead content of calcium supplements. *JAMA.* 2000;284:1425–1429.

56. Heaney, RP. Lead in calcium supplements: Cause for alarm or celebration? *JAMA.* 2000;284:1432–1433.

57. Marcus, D, and Grollman, AP. Botanical medicines: The need for new regulations. *New Engl J Med.* 2002;347,25:2073–2075.

58. Ibid.

59. Harkey, MR, et al. Variability in commercial ginseng products: An analysis of 25 preparations. *Am J Clin Nutrition.* 2001;73:1001–1006.

60. Gilroy, CM, et al. Echinacea and truth in labeling. *Arch Intern Med.* 2003; 163:699–704.

61. web.lexis-nexis.com.

62. Morris, CA, and Avorn, J. Op cit.

63. *Complementary and Alternative Medicine in the United States.* 2005. Institute of Medicine. www.nap.edu.

64. Zhang, X. *Regulatory Situation of Herbal Medicines: A Worldwide Review.* WHO. 1998. www.who.int/medicines/library/trm/who-trm-98-1.

65. Cohen, PJ. Science, politics, and the regulation of dietary supplements: It's time to repeal DSHEA. *Am J Law Med.* 2005;31:175–214.

66. Palmer, ME, et al. Adverse events associated with dietary supplements: An observational study. *Lancet.* 2003;361:101–106.

67. Lipman, MM. Herbal medicine (correspondence). *New Engl J Med.* 2003; 348:1498–1500.

## CHAPTER 9: SILICONE BREAST IMPLANTS: MISCONCEPTIONS, MISINTERPRETATIONS, AND MISTAKES

1. *Hopkins v. Dow Corning Corp.* No. C-91-2132. U.S. District Court. (1991).

2. Dore, ME. A commentary on the use of epidemiological evidence in demonstrating cause-in-fact. *Harvard Environ Law Rev* 429. 1983.

3. *Reference Manual on Scientific Evidence.* 2nd ed. Federal Judicial Center. 2001.

4. *Frye v. United States*, 293 F. 1013 (D.C. Cir. 1923).

5. Giannelli, PC. The admissibility for novel scientific evidence: Frye v. United States, a half century later. *80 Columbia Law Review.* 1980;1197:1224–1225.

6. *Daubert v. Merrell Dow Pharmaceuticals* 509 U.S. 579 (1993).

7. Huber, PW. *Galileo's Revenge: Junk Science in the Courtroom.* New York: Basic Books, 1991.

8. Rosenbaum, JT. Lessons from litigation over silicone breast implants: A call for activism by scientists. *Science.* 1997;276:1524–1525.

9. *Safety of Silicone Breast Implants.* Washington, DC: Institute of Medicine, National Academy Press, 1999.

10. Ibid.

11. Committees on Toxicity Mutagenicity and Carcinogenicity of Chemicals in Food, Consumer Products, and the Environment. *1994 Annual Report.* London: UK Department of Health, 1995.

12. VanNunen, SA, et al. Post mammoplasty connective tissue disease. *Arthritis Rheum.* 1982;25:694–697.

13. Spiera, H. Scleroderma after silicone augmentation mammoplasty. *JAMA.* 1988;260:236–238.

14. The Report of the Independent Review Group. *Silicone Gel Implants.* London: Crown Press, 1998.

15. Baines, CJ, et al. Summary of the report on silicone gel-filled breast implants. *Can Med Assoc J.* 1992;147:1141–1146.

16. *Agence Nationale Pour Le Development de L'Evaluation Medicale Les Implants Mammaires Rempllis del Gel de Silicone.* Paris: ANDEM, 1996.

17. Angell, M. *Science on Trial: The Clash of Medical Evidence and the Law in the Breast Implant Case.* New York: Norton, 1996.

18. Hennekens, CH, et al. Self-reported breast implants and connective tissue diseases in female health professionals. *JAMA.* 1996;275:616–620.

19. Janowsky, EC, et al. Meta-analysis of the relation between silicone breast implants and the risk of connective tissue diseases. *New Engl J Med* Med. 2000; 342:781–790.

20. *Safety of Silicone Breast Implants.* Institute of Medicine. Op cit.

21. *The Report of the Independent Review Group.* Op cit.

22. Fumento, M. *Silicone Breast Implants: Why Has Science Been Ignored?* New York: American Council on Science and Health, 1996.

23. *Safety of Silicone Breast Implants.* Institute of Medicine. Op cit.

24. *Food and Drug Administration Backgrounder.* No. BG 91-6. August 1, 1991.

25. Ferguson, JH. Silicone breast implants and neurological disorders—report of the Practice Committee of the American Academy of Neurology. *Neurology.* 1997; 48:1504–1507.

26. *The Report of the Independent Review Group.* Op cit.

27. Berlin, CM. Silicon breast implants and breastfeeding. *Breast Feeding Abstracts.* 1996;15:17–18.

28. Bejarano, MA, and Zimmerman, MA. *Determination of the Low Levels of Silicones in Human Breast Milk by Aqueous Silanol Functionality Test.* Dow Corning File No. 1991-1000-36332. 1991.

29. Rosenbaum, JT. Op cit.

30. *Hall v. Baxter Healthcare Corp.* 9477 F Supp. 1387 (D. Ore. 1996).

31. *General Electric Co. v. Joiner.* 118 S. Ct. 512 (1997).

32. Rosenbaum, JT. Op cit.

33. Kessler, DA. The basis of the FDA's decision on breast implants. *New Engl J Med.* 1992;326:1713–1715.

34. Angell, M. Op cit.

35. FDA rejects silicone breast implant request. CNN. January 8, 2004.

36. Peck, P. FDA allows return of silicone-gel breast implants. *MedPage Today.* November 20, 2006. www.medpagetoday.com.

37. Federal panel debates silicone breast implants. Associated Press. April 12, 2005.

## CHAPTER 10: OBESITY AND PUBLIC POLICY

1. Kersh, R, and Morone, J. The politics of obesity: Seven steps to government action. *Politics and Public Health.* 2002;21:142–153.

2. Critser, G. *Fat Land: How Americans Became the Fattest People in the World.* Boston: Houghton Mifflin, 2003.

3. Weight Control. *What Works and Why.* Medical Essay. Supplement to the Mayo Clinic Health Letter. Rochester, MN: Mayo Foundation for Medical Education and Research, 2006.

4. Satcher, D. *Surgeon General's Call to Action to Prevent and Decrease Overweight and Obesity.* Washington, DC: Department of Health and Human Services, 2001.

5. Nestle, M. The ironic politics of obesity. *Science.* 2003;299(5608):781.

6. Ibid.

7. Mei, Z, et al. Validity and body mass index compared with other body-composition screening indexes for the assessment of body fatness in children and adolescents. *Am J Clin Nutr.* 2002;75:978–985.

8. National Center for Health Statistics. Centers for Disease Control and Prevention.

9. Flegal, KM, et al. Excess deaths associated with underweight, overweight, and obesity. *JAMA.* 2005;293:1861–1867.

10. Allison, DB, et al. Annual deaths attributable to obesity in the United States. *JAMA.* 1999;282:1530–1538.

11. Caterson, ID, et al. AHA Conference Proceedings. Prevention Conference VII. Obesity, A worldwide epidemic related to health disease and stroke. Group III. Worldwide comorbidities of obesity. *Circulation.* 2004;110:476–483.

12. Must, A, et al. The disease burden associated with overweight and obesity. *JAMA.* 1999;282:1523–1529.

13. *Obesity: Preventing and Managing the Global Epidemic.* WHO Technical Report Series 894. Geneva: WHO, 2000.

14. Visscher, TLS, et al. Obesity and unhealthy life-years in adult Finns. An empirical approach. *Arch Intern Med.* 2004;164:1413–1420.

15. Chan, JM, et al. Obesity, fat distribution, and weight gain as risk factors for clinical diabetes in men. *Diabetes Care.* 1994;17:961–969.

16. Colditz, GA, et al. Weight gain as a risk factor for clinical diabetes mellitus in women. *Ann Intern Med.* 1995;122:481–486.

17. Ibid.

18. Ford, ES, et al. Weight change and diabetes incidence: Findings from a national cohort of U.S. adults. *American J Epidemiol.* 1997;146:214–222.

19. Lee, RE, and Cubbin, C. Neighborhood context and youth cardiovascular health behaviors. *Am J Public Health.* 2002;92:428–436.

20. Stern, MP, and Braxton, DM. Diabetes in Hispanic Americans. *Diabetes in America,* 2nd ed. Bethesda, MD: National Institute of Diabetes and Digestive and Kidney Diseases, 1997. www.diabetes.niddk.nih.gov/dm/pubs/america.

21. Kleinfield, NP. Living at an epicenter of diabetes, defiance, and despair. *New York Times.* January 10, 2006.

22. Morland, K, et al. Neighborhood characteristics associated with the location of food stores and food service places. *Am J Prev Med.* 2002;22:23–29.

23. *How Obesity Policies Are Failing in America.* 2005. Trust for American's Health. www.healthamericans.org.

24. Serdula, MK, et al. Do obese children become obese adults? A review of the literature. *Prev Med.* 1993;22:167–177.

25. Freedman, DS, et al. Relationship of childhood obesity to coronary heart disease risk factors in adulthood: The Bogalusa Heart Study. *Pediatrics.* 2001;108:712–718.

26. Guo, SS, et al. The predictive value for childhood body mass index values for overweight at age 35 years. *Amer J Clin Nutr.* 1994;59:810–819.

27. American Diabetes Association: Type 2 Diabetes in children and adolescents (consensus statement). *Diabetes Care.* 2000;23:381–389.

28. Flegal, KM, et al. Prevalence and trends in obesity among U.S. adults, 1999–2000. *JAMA.* 2002;288:1723–1727.

29. Ogden, CL, et al. Prevalence and trends in overweight among U.S. children and adolescents, 1999–2000. *JAMA.* 2002;288:1728–1732.

30. Ogden, CL, et al. Prevalence of overweight and obesity in the United States, 1999–2000. *JAMA.* 2006;295:1549–1555.

31. Adams, KF, et al. Overweight, obesity, and mortality in a large prospective cohort of persons 50–71 years old. *New Engl J Med.* 2006;355:763780.

32. Gerrior, S, and Bente, L. The U.S. food supply series, 1970 to 1994: Nutrient availability and policy implications. *Family Economics and Nutrition Review.* Summer 1997.

33. Malik, VS, Schulze, MB, and Hu, FB. Intake of sugar-sweetened beverages and weight gain: A systematic review. *Amer J Clin Nutr.* 2006;84:274–288.

34. Guthrie, JF, and Morton, JF. Food sources of added sweeteners in the diets of Americans. *J Amer Diet Assoc.* 2000;100:43–51.

35. Popkin, BM, and Nielsen, SJ. The sweetening of the world's diet. *Obesity Research.* 2003;11:1325–1332.

36. Kantor, LA. *A Dietary Assessment of the U.S. Food Supply: Comparing Per Capita Food Consumption with Food Guide Pyramid Service Recommendations.* U.S. Department of Agriculture. Washington, DC: Government Printing Office, 1998.

37. Johnson, RK, and Frary, C. Choose beverages and foods to moderate your intake of sugars: The 2000 dietary guidelines for Americans—what's all the fuss about? *J Nutrition.* 2001;131:2766S–2771S.

38. *2005 Dietary Guidelines for Americans.* Washington, DC: Departments of Health and Human Services and of Agriculture, 2005. www.health.gov/dietaryguidelines.

39. Prentice, RL, et al. Low-fat dietary pattern and risk of invasive breast cancer: The Women's Health Initiative Randomized Controlled Dietary Modification Trial. *JAMA.* 2006;295:629–642.

40. Warner, M. The war over salt. *New York Times.* September 13, 2006. p. C1.

41. Havas, S, Roccella, EJ, and Lenfant, C. Reducing the public health burden from elevated blood pressure levels in the United States by lowering intake of dietary sodium. *Am J Public Health.* 2004;94:19–22.

42. Nestle, M. *The Ironic Politics of Obesity.* Op cit.

43. Sims, LD. *The Politics of Fat: Food and Nutrition Policy in America.* Armonk, NY: Sharpe, 1998.

44. Ippolito, PM, and Mathios, AD. Information and advertising: The case for fat consumption in the United States. *Amer Economic Rev.* 1995;85:91–95.

45. Cawley, J. An economic framework for understanding physical activity and eating behaviors. *Amer J Prev Med.* 2004;27(S):117–125.

46. French, SA. Pricing effects of food choices. The American Society for Nutritional Sciences. *J Nutrition.* 2003;133:841S–843S.

47. French, SA, et al. Pricing and promotion effects on low-fat vending snack purchases: The HCIPS study. *Am J Public Health.* 2001;91:112–117.

48. French, SA, et al. Pricing strategy to promote fruit and vegetable purchase in high school cafeterias. *J Amer Dietetic Assn.* 1997;97:1008–1010.

49. Hill, JO, et al. Obesity and the environment: Where do we go from here? *Science.* 2003;299:853–855.

50. Nestle, M. *The Ironic Politics of Obesity.* Op cit.

51. French, SA, et al. Environmental influences on eating and physical activity. *Annual Rev Public Health.* 2001;22:309–335.

52. Nestle, M. Increasing portion sizes in American diets: More calories, more obesity. *J Amer Dietetic Assn.* 2003;103:39–40.

53. Kersh, R, and Morone, J. *The Politics of Obesity: Seven Steps to Government Action.* Op cit.

54. Mello, M, et al. Obesity—the new frontier of public health law. *New Engl J Med.* 2006;354:2601–2608.

55. Groom, N. McDonald's throws weight behind obesity research. Reuters. September 18, 2006.

56. Oliver, JE, and Lee, T. Public opinion and the politics of obesity in America. *J Health Politics, Policy and Law.* 2005;30:923–954.

57. Cleland, R, et al. *Commercial Weight Loss Products and Programs: What Consumers Stand to Gain and Lose.* Washington, DC: Federal Trade Commission, Bureau of Consumer Protection, 1998.

58. Bravata, DM, et al. Efficacy and safety of low-carbohydrate diets: A systematic review. *JAMA.* 2003;289:1837–1850.

59. Foster, GD, et al. A randomized trial of a low carbohydrate diet for obesity. *New Engl J Med.* 2003;348:2082–2091.

60. Dansinger, ML, et al. Comparison of the Atkins, Ornish, Weight Watchers, and Zone Diets for weight loss and heart disease risk reduction: A randomized trial. *JAMA.* 2005;293:43–53.

61. Goetz, T. 75 million Americans may have something called metabolic syndrome. How big pharma turned obesity into a disease then invented the drugs to cure it. *Wired.* October 2006. pp. 152–157.

62. Ibid.

63. Davidson, MH, et al. Weight control and risk factor reduction in obese patients treated for 2 years with Orlistat. *JAMA.* 1999;281:235–242.

64. Chanoine, J, et al. Effect of Orlistat on weight and body composition in obese adolescents. *JAMA.* 2005;293:2873–2883.

65. Wadden, T, et al. Randomized trial of lifestyle modifications and pharmacotherapy for obesity. *New Engl J Med.* 2005;353:2111–2120.

66. Personal Responsibility in Food Consumption Act. 108th Congress. 2nd session. HR 339.

67. Boseley, S. United States accused of sabotaging obesity strategy. *Internatl J Health Services.* 2004;34:553–554.

68. Connolly, C. Public policy targeting obesity. *Washington Post.* August 10, 2003. p. A1.

69. Kersh, R, and Morone, J. How the personal becomes political: Prohibitions, public health, and obesity. *Studies in American Political Development.* 2002;16:162–175.

70. Jacobson, MF, and Brownell, KD. Small taxes on soft drinks and snack foods to promote health. *Am J Public Health.* 2000;90:854–856.

71. Ibid.

72. Oliver, JE, and Lee, T. Op cit.

73. *State Actions to Promote Nutrition, Increase Physical Activity, and Prevent Obesity. A 2006 First Quarter Legislative Overview.* NetScan's Health Policy Tracking Service. www.rwjf.org.

74. *A Lot Easier Said than Done: Parents Talk About Raising Children in Today's America. Public Agenda.* 2002. www.publicagenda.org.

75. *Bipartisan Support on Capitol Hill for Healthier School Foods.* Center for Science in the Public Interest. www.cspinet.org.

76. Child Nutrition Promotion and School Lunch Protection Act of 2006. 109th Congress. 2nd session.

77. Caballero, B, et al. Pathways: A school-based, randomized controlled trial for the prevention of obesity in American Indian schoolchildren. *Amer J Clin Nutr.* 2003;78:1030–1038.

78. Luepker, RV, et al. Outcomes of a field trial to improve children's dietary patterns and physician activity: The Child and Adolescent Trial for Cardiovascular Health (CATCH). *JAMA.* 1996;275:768–776.

79. Gortmaker, SL, et al. Impact of a school-based interdisciplinary intervention on diet and physical activity among urban primary school children. *Arch Pediatric Adolesc Med.* 1999;153:975–983.

80. Sallis, JF, et al. The effects of a 2-year physical education program (SPARK) on physical activity and fitness in elementary school students. *Am J Public Health.* 1997;87:1328–1334.

81. Gortmaker, SL, et al. Reducing obesity via a school-based interdisciplinary intervention among youth: Planet health. *Arch Pediatric Adolesc Med.* 1999;153:409–418.

82. Robinson, TH. Reducing children's television viewing to prevent obesity. *JAMA.* 1999;282:1561–1567.

83. Belkin, L. The school lunch test. *New York Times Magazine.* August 20, 2006. pp. 30–35, 48, 52–55.

84. *State Actions to Promote Nutrition, Increase Physical Activity, and Prevent Obesity.* Op cit.

85. Ibid.

## CHAPTER 11: DISEASE PREVENTION THROUGH VACCINATION: THE SCIENCE AND THE CONTROVERSY

1. Barquest, N, and Domingo, P. Smallpox: The triumph over the most terrible of the ministers of death. *Annals Internal Med.* 1997;127:627.

2. U.S. Centers for Disease Control and Prevention. *Ten Great Public Health Achievements in the Twentieth Century, 1900–1999.* www.cdc.gov/od/co/media/tengpha.htm.

3. Parker, AA. Implications of a 2005 measles outbreak in Indiana for sustained elimination of measles in the United States. *New Engl J Med.* 2006;355:1184.

4. Okonek, BAM, and Peters, PM. *Vaccines—How and Why.* www.access excellence.org.

5. Baxby, D. *Vaccination: Jenner's Legacy.* Berkeley, United Kingdom: Jenner Educational Trust, 1994.

6. Parish, HJ. *A History of Immunization.* Edinburgh: Livingstone, 1965.

7. Gross, CP, and Sepkowitz, K. The myth of the medical breakthrough: Smallpox, vaccination, and Jenner reconsidered. *Internatl J Infect Dis.* 1998;3:54–60.

8. Parish, HJ. Op cit.

9. Salmon, DA, et al. Compulsory vaccination and conscientious or philosophical exemptions: Past, present, and future. *Lancet.* 2006;367(9508):436–442.

10. Hansen, B. America's first medical breakthrough: How popular excitement about a French rabies cure in 1885 raised new expectations for medical progress. *American Historical Rev.* 1998;103:373–418.

11. *Smallpox.* World Health Organization. www.who.int.

12. Payette, PJ, and Davis, HL. History of vaccines and positioning of current trends. *Current Drug Targets Infectious Disorders.* 2001;1:241–247.

13. Cody, CL, et al. Nature and rates of adverse reactions associated with DPT and DT immunizations in infants and children. *Pediatrics.* 1981;68:650–660.

14. Hennessen, W, and Quest, U. Adverse reactions after pertussis vaccination. International Symposium on Immunization: Benefits vs. Risk Factors. *Brussels Developments in Biological Standardization.* 1979;43:95–100.

15. Hinman, AAR, and Koplan, J. Pertussis and pertussis vaccine: Reanalysis of benefits, risks, and costs. *JAMA.* 1984;251:3109–3113.

16. Institute of Medicine. *DPT Vaccine and Chronic Nervous System Dysfunction: A New Analysis.* Washington, DC: National Academy of Sciences, 1999.

17. Alderslade R, et al. The National Childhood Encephalopathy Study: A report on 1000 cases of serious neurological disorders in infants and young children from the NCES research team. In Department of Health and Social Security. *Whooping Cough: Reports from the Committee on the Safety of Medicines and the Joint Committee on Vaccination and Immunisation.* London: Her Majesty's Stationery Office, 1981.

18. Blume, S, and Geesink, I. Essay on science and society: A brief history of polio vaccines. *Science*. 2000;288(5471):1593–1594.

19. Biddle, W. *A Field Guide to Germs*. New York: Henry Holt, 1995.

20. Durbach, N. They might as well brand us: Working-class resistance to compulsory vaccination in Victorian England. *Social History of Medicine*. 2000;13:45–62.

21. Ibid.

22. Beck, A. Issues in the anti-vaccination movement in England. *Medical History*. 1960;4:310–321.

23. Colgrove, J. Bodily matters: The anti-vaccination movement in England. *J Health Politics Policy and Law*. 2006;31:864–867.

24. Salmon, DA, et al. Op cit.

25. Wolfe, RM, and Sharp, LK. Anti-vaccinationists past and present. *BMJ*. 2002; 325:430–432.

26. Kaufman, M. The American anti-vaccination leagues. *Archives of Disease in Childhood*. 1984:59:1195–1196.

27. Ibid.

28. Salmon, DA, et al. Op cit.

29. Goodman, R, et al. (eds.). *Law in Public Health Practice*. Oxford: Oxford University Press, 2003.

30. Salmon, DA, et al. Op cit.

31. Orenstein, WA, and Hinman, AR. The immunization system in the United States: The role of school immunization laws. *Vaccine*. 1999;17(Suppl 3):S19–S24.

32. Salmon, DA, et al. Op cit.

33. Orenstein, WA, and Hinman, AR. Op cit.

34. Measles and school immunization requirements—United States. *MMWR*. 1978;27:303–304.

35. Omer, SB, et al. Nonmedical exemptions to school immunization requirements. Secular trends and association of state policies with pertussis incidence. JAMA. 2006;296:1757–1763.

36. Salmon, DA, et al. Exemptions to school immunization requirements: The role of school-level requirements, policies, and procedures. *Am J Public Health*. 2005;95:436–440.

37. Chen, R, et al. Investigation of a possible association between influenza vaccination and Guillain-Barré syndrome in the United States, 1990–1991. *Post-Marketing Surveillance*. 1992;6:5.

38. Kaker, JP. The pertussis vaccine controversy in Great Britain, 1974–1986. *Vaccine*. 2003;21:4003–4010.

39. Meszaros, JR, et al. Cognitive processes and the decisions of some parents to forgo pertussis vaccination for their children. *J Clin Epidemiol*. 1996;49:697–703.

40. Petousis-Harris, H, et al. Family physician perspectives on barriers to childhood immunization. *Vaccine*. 2004;22:2340–2344.

41. Gellin, BG, Mailbach, EW, and Marcuse, EK. Do parents understand immunizations? A national telephone survey. *Pediatrics*. 2000;106:1097–1102.

42. Offit, PA, et al. Addressing parents' concerns: Do multiple vaccines overwhelm or weaken the infant's immune system? *Pediatrics*. 2002;109:124–129.

43. Abbott, VP. Web page quality: Can we measure it and what do we find? A report of exploratory findings. *J Public Health Med*. 2000;22:191–197.

44. Zimmerman, RK, et al. Vaccine criticism on the World Wide Web. *J Med Internet Research.* 2005;7:2.

45. Wakefield, AJ, et al. Ileal-lymphoid-nodular hyperplasia, nonspecific colitis, and pervasive developmental disorder in children. *Lancet.* 1998;351(9130):637–641.

46. Nicoll, A, Elliman, D, and Ross, E. MMR vaccinations and autism 1998. *BMJ.* 1998;316:715–716.

47. Institute of Medicine. *Immunization Safety Review: Measles-Mumps-Rubella Vaccine and Autism.* Washington, DC: National Academy Press, 2001.

48. Institute of Medicine. *Vaccines and Autism.* Washington, DC: National Academy Press, 2004.

49. Subcommittee on Human Rights and Wellness, Committee about Reform. U.S. House of Representatives. The Congressional Record. May 21, 2003.

50. Institute of Medicine. 1999. Op cit.

51. Folb, PI, et al. A global perspective on vaccine safety and public health: The Global Advisory Committee on Vaccine Safety. *Am J Public Health.* 2004;94:1926–1931.

52. McNeil, DG. Malaria vaccine proves effective. *New York Times.* October 15, 2004.

53. Grady, D. Before shortage of flu vaccine, many warnings. *New York Times.* October 17, 2004.

54. Stern, AM, and Markel, H. The history of vaccines and immunization: Familiar patterns, new challenges. *Health Affairs.* 2005;24:611–621.

# Index

# About the Author and Contributors

MADELON LUBIN FINKEL is a professor of clinical public health at the Weill Medical College of Cornell University. She serves as director of the Office of Global Health Education as well as director of Cornell Analytics Consulting Services at Weill Medical College. Health care policy and women's health issues are the focus of her research. She has written scores of scientific papers and also authored *Understanding the Mammography Controversy: Science, Politics, and Breast Cancer Screening* (Praeger, 2005). This is her tenth book on issues in health care.

RYAN CAULEY is a second-year medical student at the Weill Medical College of Cornell University. He graduated from Bowdoin College in 2003 with a degree in biology. He has worked at the University of California–Berkeley's School of Public Health and with the Epilepsy Family Study at Columbia University's Mailman School of Public Health. He recently spent a summer at the University of Cape Town Medical School working on both HIV and transplant surgery.

SANDRA M. DEMARS is a second-year medical student at the Weill Medical College of Cornell University. A native of Ridgefield, Connecticut, she graduated from the University of Texas–Austin in 2001 with a BS in biochemistry. From 2001 to 2003 she was a medical researcher at Rockefeller University focusing on the genetics of schizophrenia. From 2003 to 2005 she worked in a laboratory at the Tufts University School of Medicine, researching cancer signal transduction. She also spent a summer in Durban, South Africa, working in various types of HIV/AIDS medical care settings with Child Family Health International.

IVAN IP is a fourth-year medical student at the Weill Medical College of Cornell University. After completing his undergraduate degree in chemical engineering in 2001, he became involved in public health, with a particular interest in health policy, outcomes research, and environmental health. He served as an AmeriCorps Fellow for two years and became an active advocate for the uninsured population in his local community. He earned his MPH from the University of California–Berkeley.

TONY ROSEN is a first-year medical student at the Weill Medical College of Cornell University. Previously, he studied epidemiology and earned his MPH at UCLA, concentrating in methodology and questionnaire design and access.